Table of Contents

In conclusion

Introduction

Is Intermittent Fasting a good thing?

"Isn't breakfast the most substantial meal of the day?"

"Want to lose weight? Make sure you start your day with a healthy breakfast so that your metabolism starts working. Have your breakfast like kings, lunch as princes, and dinner as poor. "

"Want to lose more weight? Try to eat six little meals a day, so that your body works at maximum capacity all day long. "

Nowadays, we discover so much about the importance of starting the day early and breakfast for healthy living and weight control. There are even studies showing that those who consume the first meal early in the day lose more weight than those who consume the first meal late or skip meals. So when you start your day with breakfast, do you get healthier or lose more weight?

But with a sceptical approach can we ask the question: what if there is scientific research that shows that skipping breakfast is more effective for optimum efficiency, maximum muscle involvement and fat loss?

Intermittent fasting, i.e. intermittent fasting is not a diet; is a nutrition scheme. In other words, it is based on an informed decision to skip certain meals. Intermittent fasting based on consciously starving before a certain period after eating; it means choosing to eat your meals at certain times of the day (eating window) and not to eat at rest times (hunger window).

It is not easy to define the concept of Intermittent fasting because there are many different ways to implement it correctly. Intermittent fasting is practiced in different concepts around the world. The usual common versions of intermittent fasting are:

1. Fasting every other day: Fasting every other day, as the name suggests, is the name given to fasting every two days. Nothing is invincible on fasting days, that is, hunger windows, while on other days, an average of around 500 calories is eaten.
2. The Warrior Diet: The Warrior Diet, also known as this method the only day in food in large portions at dinner defeat of fruits and vegetables is based on the defeat.
3. Fasting 16/8: When practicing 16/8, fasting is carried out 16 hours a day, and the eating window is fitted to the remaining 8 hours. Often, after dinner and eat the next day in the morning, breakfast is applied by skipping.
4. Ye-Dur-Ye: It is practiced 24 hours a day or two of the week by not eating anything. The rest of the week is free of nutrition.
5. 5: 2 diet: 5: 2 concept, 5 days a week while eating normal, the remaining two days of calorie intake is based on keeping between 500-600 calories.

How intermittent fasting is applied?

➢ Regularly eating at a specific time interval: for example, eating only between the hour of 12:00 and 20:00 and skipping breakfast, some people who apply intermittent fasting can leave this interval for 6 hours or even 4 hours.

>   Skipping two meals a day and not eating anything 24 hours a day: for example, having your dinner in your normal order and not eating anything until dinner the next day.

After the above explanations, the working logic of intermittent fasting may look like this; I'm I skipped meals and had less food in total. Therefore I will give more weight." This is partly true. By eliminating any meal, even if you eat more of your other meals, the total amount of calories you receive is reduced, and you are getting closer to losing weight. However, since not all calories have the same effect on the body, the hour you eat can change your body's response to calories.

How does intermittent fasting work?

When you perform intermittent fasting, your body works in different ways during times of hunger and satiety:

When you eat, your body processes and burns what you eat for several hours. Since the foods you eat give the body the materials it can burn to produce energy; the body uses what you consume as a source of energy, not the stored oil. This is especially true if you consume carbohydrates or sugars; because the body prefers to use sugar before any source.

In the hunger window, since the body does not have a recently consumed food source for use in energy production, it is directed to the fats stored in your body rather than sugar in the bloodstream or glycogen in the muscle and liver.

Burn fat = gain.

The fact that your body uses fat stored for energy also applies when you are doing sports while you are on hunger. Unable to find a ready source of glucose or glycogen, the body has to use its only energy source: fats stored in your cells.

So how does this work? The body responds to food by producing insulin. The more sensitive your body is to insulin, the more effective it is to use the nutrients you consume; therefore, it supports fat burning and muscle formation, on the other hand, when your body is most sensitive to insulin, the time after the hunger process.

The glycogen in your body (starch stored in your muscles/liver and used by the body as a fuel when it is needed) decreases during sleep, i.e. hunger; during physical activity, it decreases even further and insulin sensitivity increases. So the food you consume right after the sport is stored most effectively: a large part as glycogen in your muscles, a part as energy for use in healing and resting, and a small amount as fat.

To compare this to a day when you don't use intermittent fasting: when your insulin sensitivity is at normal levels, carbohydrates and foods you consume to fill up your glycogen stores, the quantity of glucose in your blood reaches a sufficient level, and so most of what you eat is stored as fat. On the other hand, growth hormone secretion increases during fasting (both during sleep and at the end of hunger windows). Increased secretion of growth hormone, decreased insulin production and consequently increased insulin sensitivity while applying intermittent fasting, the body is ready for muscle development and fat loss.

To put it differently: Intermittent fasting helps your body teach you to use the nutrients it consumes more efficiently. For many different physiological reasons, when applied correctly, intermittent fasting accelerates weight loss and muscle formation.

So why do all health books recommend eating 6 6 meals a day?

Here are the reasons why many nutrition and diet books recommend eating 6 meals a day:

1. When you eat, your body system has to burn extra calories to process the foods you consume. The theory works as follows; if you eat small meals all day long, your body regularly burns extra calories; your metabolism also works at the optimum capacity. However, this information is not correct. Whether you consume 2000 calories in a short time

     or broadcast all day; your body consumes the same amount of calories when processing these foods. Although the proposal to increase your metabolism rate by eating continuously seems to work in theory, it is unfortunately in practice in the classroom.

2. When you make your meals more frequent and smaller, your chances of over-eating your main meals are reduced. Although this information is partially correct; it is not necessary to eat six meals a day as long as you teach yourself portion control or control what you eat. On the other hand, you'll probably never feel full when you eat 6 small meals, and so your chances of turning your snacks to higher calorie options will increase.

In short, 6 meals a day does not work in practice, as it does not work at the point where you think it works.

Returning to the Stone Age; it was not possible for our ancestors to eat every 3 hours under the conditions they lived in that period. Our ancestors were only fed when they found food, and even in this case, their body had adapted to work all day.

A recent study published in the New York Times discussed the technique of verme losing weight by eating 6 meals a day". According to Martin, one of the writers of Lean Gains, the most important implications of the research are as follows:

The suggestion of the study was to increase the frequency of eating by providing short-term hunger control and increasing the likelihood of dieting; furthermore, the predicted beneficial effects of increasing the frequency of eating were that it provided better intestinal peptides and thus greater weight loss. All three hypotheses were refuted under the conditions given in the research."

"It was accepted that increased food frequency would increase the likelihood of adhering to energy-restricting diets and, therefore, would facilitate weight loss with increased satiety. However, the results do not confirm this hypothesis. "

Remember what you eat is essential. Eating frequency; the amount you eat and the quality of the food you eat are not as important.

Why Intermittent Fasting?

- Because it works, not all calories taken affect the body in the same way; however, calorie restriction is one of the cornerstones of losing weight. When you practice intermittent fasting, whichever method you choose, you also make it easier to restrict the number of calories you take during the week. You are less likely to lose weight because you have received fewer calories than before.
- Because it makes your job easier, instead of feeding 6 small meals a day, you don't have to try to pack, pack and eat every 2-3 hours.
- Because it takes less time and money, you spend only 3-6 meals a day, while you spend less and less time and money for 3-6 meals a day, and you only spend 2 meals a day at intermittent fasting.
- Because it supports muscle gain and weight loss, intermittent fasting increases insulin sensitivity and growth hormone secretion, which are the cornerstones of muscle development.

Intermittent fasting is not a common side effect of intermittent fasting. Many people worry about intermittent fasting, the lack of energy that long-term hunger can cause, loss of focus and the feeling of hunger. The number of people, who think that energy will drop during the day, especially when skipping breakfast, isn't much less.

The first time you switch from eating throughout the day to intermittent fasting, your body may have a little strain. However, when you complete the transition process, your body will quickly adjust to the new order and work as well as the order you eat throughout the day. In a study examining participants during and at the end of a 48-hour fasting window, it was concluded that 2 cognitive performance, activity, sleep and psychological state were not adversely affected in 2-day calorie deficiency in healthy individuals".

"Why do not I feel grumpy breakfast well?" She asks if you will; maybe you're eating habits are the reason for your crankiness. The body, used to eating at frequent intervals, will wait for you to eat every 3 hours, as learning. In other words, if you have breakfast every morning, your body will ask you to have breakfast every morning when it wakes up. We can say that this process has both physical and psychological origins.

If you re-train your body so that it does not expect to eat every day or throughout the day; with ghrelin hormone secretion, side effects will become less effective. Returning to the cave era, our ancestors were able to survive periods of abundance as well as periods of famine. Remember, long-term starvation requires 84 hours to modify glucose levels in the body negatively. So 16 or 24-hour hunger windows are not a time your body can't handle.

Important warning:

Intermittent fasting; It can be a challenging process for people with conditions such as blood sugar problems, hypoglycemia, diabetes. If you have any discomfort, you should consult your doctor or dietitian before starting intermittent fasting.

Can I develop muscle or gain weight during intermittent fasting?

Exactly! Steve Kamb applies intermittent fasting in the bodybuilding process; muscles while developing the body fat ratio in a small amount of the same amount of calories in this process while taking calories in the 8-hour windows underlines. As for the program:

> 11 AM - Heavy strength training during fasting
> 12 PM - Consumption of ½ of daily calories immediately after sports
> 7 PM - Consuming the remaining half of your daily calories as dinner
> 8 PM - 12 PM (next day): 16-hour fast

This program, which is also included in Lean Gains, is one of the most effective programs for intermittent fasting. According to another program by

Nate Green, you can effectively develop muscle by holding 24-hour fasts on Sundays every week. This method also challenges the "bulk & cut" method that is commonly used in bodybuilding. Compared to intermittent fasting and the classic bulk & cut method to develop muscle, when intermittent fasting:

- Your balance does not deteriorate: So you do not need to take 30 kilograms and give 25 to get 5kg muscle. So your body mass doesn't change much.
- You eat less, so your money stays in your pocket: Instead of the weight you get, you need to consume as much muscle and fat as you need. Slowly, steadily, steadily and permanently, you gain muscle and strength.
- The concept of the holiday body does not interest you: We all want to look good, especially in the summer when the clothes are thinner and smaller. In a scenario where your muscles develop regularly, you don't have to worry about how you look at any stage of the process.

Does intermittent fasting have different effects on women and men?

Yes, intermittent fasting affects men and women differently. A writing on Paleo for Women focuses on the negative effects of intermittent fasting for women. Another article in Mark's Daily Apple highlights the differences in the male and female body and explains how they are affected by intermittent fasting:

- In one study, intermittent fasting increased insulin sensitivity in men, but not in women.

- Another study examined the effect of day-fasting on blood lipids. Triglycerides remained stable while HDL increased benign cholesterol in women; in men, HDL remained stable, while triglyceride rate decreased. Although the effect of intermittent fasting on blood lipids varies depending on gender, the results were found to be positive in both cases.
- In another study, it was seen that body fat, weight, blood pressure, cholesterol, malignant LDL cholesterol and

triglyceride rates decreased in obese women and obese men who applied intermittent fasting. It should be noted, however, that the participants were obese and that premenopausal women were excluded from the study and that these results may not be the same in weaker people or women who have not yet had menopause.

In short, intermittent fasting experiences of men and women can result in different; however, since we all have different bodies, there is nothing more natural than not having the same results as another. Therefore, to reach the most accurate information, you can try to apply a program that suits you and see with your own eyes.

Top Questions about Intermittent Fasting

One of the commonly asked questions about intermittent fasting is usually "won't I get hungry? As mentioned above, the fact that you're not hungry is all about the pattern your body is used to. If you eat something during the day, or if you have a particular hour you eat every day, your body will get used to this order and start preparing insulin for food. However, after a short period of acclimatization, your body will also accept a new order.

Remember, your body's physical and cognitive abilities are not adversely affected by fasting.

Where do I receive the energy to do sports? Will, I do not get tired if I am hungry, or will I be able to complete my workouts? After your body becomes used to the unique order, even if you don't eat before sports, it starts working as usual.

Even training on empty stomach results in better metabolic adaptation, i.e. better performance, increased muscle protein synthesis, and a greater anabolic response to post-sport food; In other words, when you do sports when you eat both you eat, and you will earn the muscles you deserve.

When doing sports, you can arrange your open window to fit your sports schedule. The crucial thing here is that if you are not an athlete who needs to perform at any moment, you should not worry and don't panic. If you only want to lose a few pounds or muscle, try to do your best.

Can fasting cause muscle loss?". This is one of the most asked questions in the mind of people who want to apply intermittent fasting. But it's a baseless concern. Because "the body's hourly protein amount of 30 grams for several hours if you do not take your body begins to use your muscles as a source of energy" is not true information.

A study shows that the body protects muscles even in the event of hunger. In other words, the body's process of protein processing can take longer than said. On the other hand, spreading the total amount of protein you need to take all day or consuming in a short time does not make any difference to your body.

So if I don't eat for a long time, will my body go through starvation?". The thought process here is as follows: Since our body thinks that we cannot get the necessary calories when we do not eat, we begin to store the limited calories you take instead of burning; therefore, the weight loss effect of starvation disappears. However, this approach is not entirely correct, either. Martin, one of the authors of Lean Gain, clarifies:

- ❖ 60 The earliest time the body recognizes hunger and lowers metabolic rate is 60 hours. According to different studies, the metabolic rate is not affected by fasting before 72-96 hours.
- ❖ On the other hand, although it may seem like a paradox, the metabolic rate rises in short-term hunger situations. To give clear figures, research has reported an increase of 3.6% to 10% in 36-48 hours of fasting.
- ❖ Epinephrine and norepinephrine (adrenaline and noradrenaline) sharpen the mind and make us active. Behavior like hunting and hunting increases the chances of survival. At some point, for example, if you don't eat for a few days, it's more advantageous if the body stores what you eat."

If your diet provides you with benefits such as muscle development, weight loss, reduction in body fat, and you are healthy, continue using the same method. However, if what you're doing isn't working, you don't get the results you want, or it makes you feel bad, you can give it a different way. Trying something new is the most effective way to know if it will do you any good.

First, Maybe in the fasting window for 15 hours instead of 16? Relax, because your body is a customizable machine and everything is not as black or white as you think. If your desire to change your diet stems from aesthetic concerns or athletic performance, of course, you should be more consistent and punctual; but in other cases, there is no point in stressing yourself.

Try to keep yourself busy. If you are sitting without doing anything and thinking about how hungry you are, the more the process will challenge you.

When applying intermittent fasting, there are a few tips that will increase your productivity and make your life easier:

- Start the hunger window immediately after a hearty meal. When you're satiated enough, the last thing you'll want to think about is eating.
- Be sure to match the 8 hours of the 16-hour fasting window to your sleep process.
- If you haven't eaten just before sleep, you'll have left behind the hunger window for about 8-12 hours. It can be operated in the last 4 hours, and you can also spend the last 1 hour.
- You can consume calorie-free drinks while in the hunger window; you can drink green tea to meet your caffeine need. If you require drinking water, black coffee or tea, do not push yourself too hard and listen to the sound of your body.

When changing your diet, do not forget to observe the changes in your body.

- If you are afraid that you will lose your muscle mass, follow your strength training program more closely.
- Be sure to measure your body fat regularly.
- Keep track of your calories; so you can closely observe how your body changes by consuming the same amount of food.

Different bodies can react differently to intermittent fasting; you will not know what your body reaction will be. Therefore, it is up to you to listen to your body and make the necessary changes during this process.

Intermittent fasting helps you lose weight while increasing your insulin sensitivity and growth hormone secretion; however, it is only one of the hundreds of factors that affect your body shape and health. Don't expect to get rid of your fat mass by just having breakfast. You should have healthy eating habits, consume more quality and healthy foods and try to get stronger. Intermittent fasting is just one of the factors that will contribute to your success.

Intermittent fasting has potential positive effects for people who want to lose weight or increase muscle mass. The male and female bodies react separately to the intermittent fasting, just as each can react differently to the same situation. So the most effective way to see if the fasting is right for you is to try.

Intermittent Fasting and Benefits: Lose Weight, Protect Your Heart and Brain

Diet is everyone's dream: to lose weight while being able to eat anything you want for most of the week, paying attention to what you only eat for a day or two. Believe it or not: intermittent fasting is not only a slimming waist; it keeps your blood sugar level in balance, reduces inflammation and protects your heart health.

Although approaches to intermittent fasting are different, many studies highlight the benefits of intermittent fasting to your health.

From fasting for several hours every day to skipping meals two days a week, intermittent fasting is one of the easiest and immediate ways to maintain your health and achieve your weight goals.

6 Benefits of Intermittent Fasting

1. Supports weight loss.

One of the most notable advantages of intermittent fasting is that it accelerates fat burning and helps you get rid of excess. One of the reasons why many people are using intermittent fasting instead of traditional diets is that you ought not to keep track of what you eat and calories constantly.

Intermittent fasting provides the use of fat stores in your body as energy, accelerating fat burning and weight loss. When you eat, your body utilizes glucose as the main source of energy and stores the remaining nutrients as glycogen in your muscles and liver. When you don't provide a regular flow of glucose to your body, the body begins to break down glycogen to use it as a source of energy. As glycogen decreases, the body starts to look for alternative energy sources and turns to fat cells.

The similarity between the intermittent fasting and the ketogenic diet is that both force your body to use oil as an energy source, depriving you of carbohydrates.

In research conducted in 2015 focusing on the effects of fasting every other day, it was concluded that this fast reduced body weight by 7% and resulted in an average loss of 4kg of fat. Similar results were achieved with all-day fasting, which resulted in a 9% reduction in body weight. However, the effects of fasting on the muscles all day have not been adequately explained.

In another study focusing on 16/8 interval fasting, it was concluded that this method significantly reduces the body fat and maintains muscle mass and strength.

2. He's regulating his blood sugar

When you eat, carbohydrates are shredded into glucose and mixed into the blood. The hormone called insulin transports glucose from the bloodstream to the cells where it will be used as energy. However, if you have diabetes, insulin doesn't always work. In this case, blood sugar rises, causing problems such as fatigue, thirst and increased toilet need.

Some research on the subject, intermittent fasting regulates blood sugar, fast ups and downs have been concluded that prevent.

In one study, participants with diabetes fasted for an average of 16 hours daily for two weeks. At the end of two weeks, it was observed that the calorie intake decreased and there was a vital decrease in blood sugar levels in addition to weight loss.

In another study, fasting reduced blood sugar by 12% as well as insulin levels were reduced by about 53%. The result of the research is as follows: Preventing insulin secretion makes insulin work more efficiently and makes your body more sensitive to the effects of insulin.

3. Protecting your heart

One of the most impressive aspects of intermittent fasting is its positive effects on heart health. Research shows that intermittent fasting protects your heart health by reducing the risk of certain heart diseases.

In one of the studies, it was concluded that intermittent fasting positively affected some of the factors supporting heart health. Intermittent fasting increases HDL cholesterol, which is known as good cholesterol and low cholesterol LDL and triglyceride rates.

In a study conducted in animals published in the Journal of Nutritional Biochemistry, it was concluded that intermittent fasting increases adiponectin levels. Adiponectin is a hormone that performs a role in fat and sugar metabolism and protects against heart disease and heart attack.

In another study, it was observed that the chances of getting rid of a heart attack in rats fed with fasting by day increased by 66% compared to rats fed with a normal diet.

4. Itihaplanını reduces.

Inflammation, the body's typical response to disability. Chronic inflammation is a condition that can lead to chronic diseases. Some studies even suggest that chronic inflammation is associated with diseases such as heart attacks, diabetes, obesity and cancer.

5. It protects your brain.

In addition to protecting your heart health and keeping you away from diseases, some research has shown that intermittent fasting also helps maintain brain health.

A study of animals has shown that intermittent fasting improves cognitive functions and protects the brain against changes in memory and learning ability. In another study on animals, it was concluded that intermittent fasting protects the brain of mice by affecting certain proteins involved in ageing the brain.

The anti-inflammatory impacts of intermittent fasting can also help slow the development of diseases such as Alzheimer's disease.

6. Reduces hunger

Leptin, also known as the fasting hormone, is a hormone produced by fat cells, signalling to stop eating. The level of leptin decreases when you are hungry, and the level of leptin increases when you start to saturate.

Since leptin is produced in fat cells, the body's leptin hormone is higher in overweight or obese people. However, high levels of circulating leptin can lead to leptin resistance and make it difficult to respond to signs of hunger.

In a study conducted with 80 participants, the researchers measured leptin levels during intermittent fasting and concluded that the amount of leptin was lower during fasting nights.

Low levels of leptin mean less leptin resistance, less hunger and more weight loss.

Warnings

Although intermittent fasting has many benefits to your health, intermittent fasting may not be the right diet for people with disorders such as gallstones, eating disorders, thyroid disorders.

For example, if your blood sugar is low, not eating all day can lower your blood sugar even further, causing tremors, heart palpitations and fatigue. If you have diabetes, you should ask your doctor before taking intermittent fasting.

If you have a history of eating disturbances, intermittent fasting may trigger past unhealthy eating symptoms. Intermittent fasting is not recommended for developmental children.

If you're sick, it's best not to take intermittent fasting so you can get the nutrients you regularly need to get better and feel better.

Pregnant women should also have a diet plan rich in vitamins and minerals, so intermittent fasting is not recommended. Since hormonal problems may occur in some women after intermittent fasting, it is beneficial to take a break from fasting on certain days of the week.

If you have gallbladder discomfort, fasting, gallbladder problems can lead to; it is recommended not to apply.

Finally, research has shown that intermittent fasting can affect thyroid hormone levels. If you have any thyroid problems, you should consult your doctor before intermittent fasting.

If you have an active life, there is no problem in doing sports while intermittent fasting? You can do sports on fasting days; however, do not force yourself too much and take care to drink plenty of water. If you have a hunger window that lasts longer than 72 hours, it is recommended that you limit your physical activity.

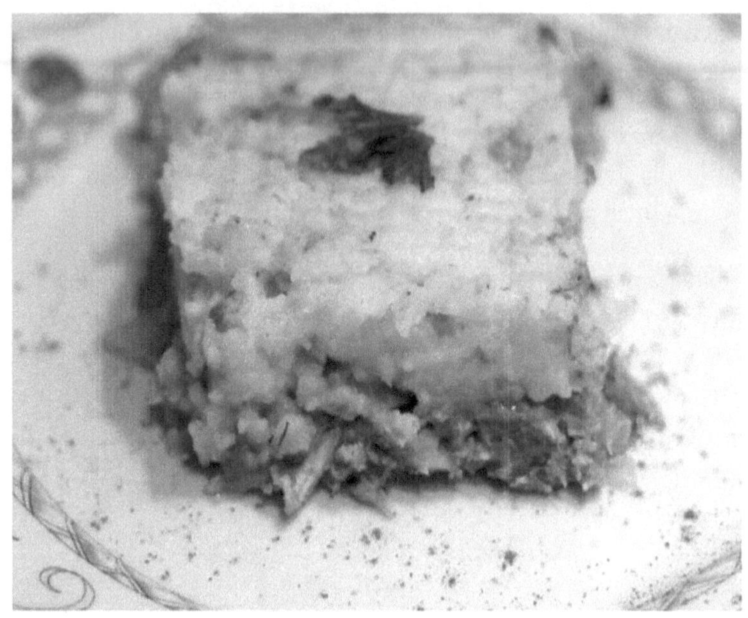

1. Chicken Pie with Chicken

A recipe without flours, ideal for making in advance and freezing

90 minutes

For 5 servings

Ingredients

One whole chicken puck

Three large potatoes (or sweet potatoes)

Two onions

Four cloves garlic

1/2 cup tomato sauce

1 cup cooked green banana puree (it is only to prepare the green banana for 8

min in the pressure cooker another option to give consistency is to use 1 cup of the milk that you like the most and two c. Of cornstarch)

One tablespoon lard

1 cup approximately milk (whichever you want)

Condiments: salt, black pepper, and cayenne, paprika, nutmeg, cumin, curry

Preparation

1.   First, cook the chicken breast in water. Prepare it in the pressure cooker and leave 20 minutes since the pot boils.

2.   Cook the chicken, prepares the potatoes in water to make the puree.

3.   Make the mash stepping potatoes with the butter and go putting the milk to give the consistency that you like. Season with salt, black pepper, and nutmeg.

4.   Now that the chicken cooled, you can crush everything tiny.

5.   In a saucepan brown the onion with a minimum of oil. Add the garlic, the tomato sauce, and the chicken. Mix well, if this medium dry adds a little water. Go putting the condiments: salt, black pepper, and cayenne, cumin, curry. Try to see if it is to your liking.

6.   If you already like how it was great. But if you want a creamier consistency, the green banana puree is ideal, if not an option is to use the milk with the cornstarch.

7.   To assemble the dish, put down the sautéed chicken and top with the mashed potatoes. Take to oven under 180 ° C for 20 minutes.

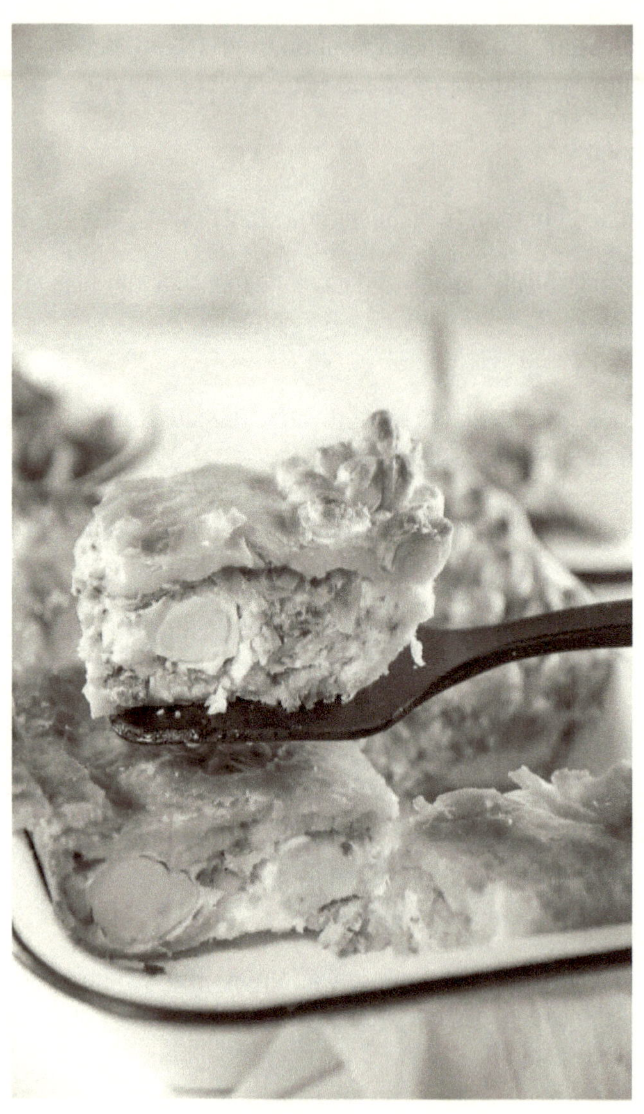

2. The classic bacon with eggs

Prep time: 10 mins

4 portions

Ingredients

8 eggs

150 g bacon, sliced

Cherry Tomato (optional)

Fresh parsley (optional)

Preparation

1. Fry the bacon until crispy. Set aside on a plate.
2. Fry the eggs in the bacon fat the way you like. Cut the cherry tomatoes in half and fry them at the same time.
3. Salt and pepper to taste.

Advice!

If you can, try using organic bacon. it's healthier and contains fewer additives.

Nutrition Facts

Ketogenic low in carbons

Per portion

Net carbohydrates: 2% (1 g)

Fiber: 0 g

Fat: 76% (23 g)

Protein: 23% (16 g)

Kcal: 282

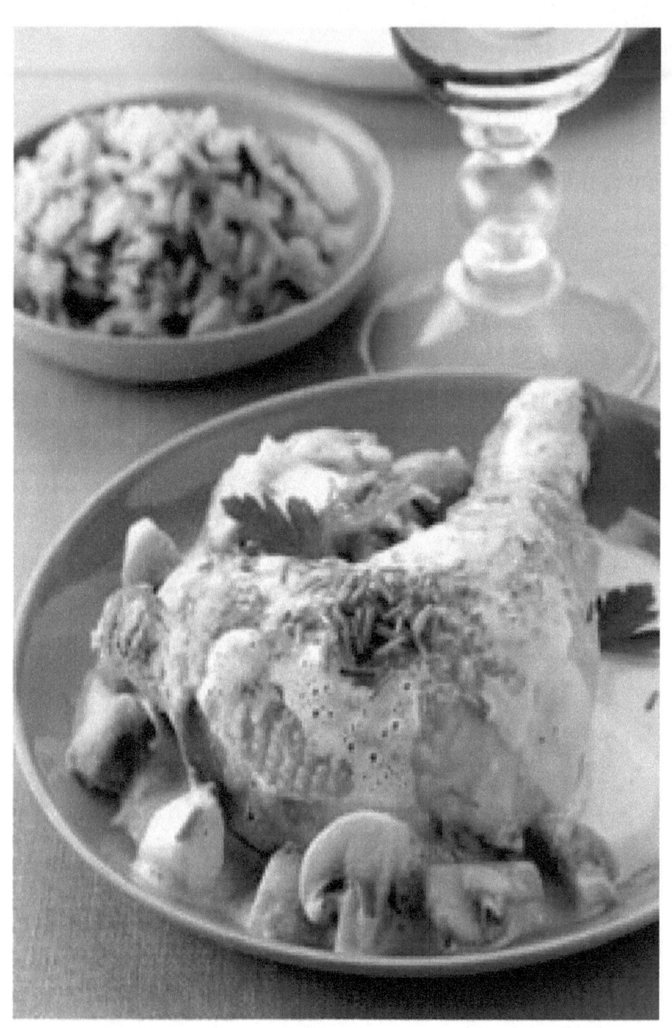

3. Hunter chicken

For: 4 people

Preparation time: 15 minutes

Cooking time: 40 minutes

Ingredients

1 whole chicken about 1.4 or 1.5 kg

300 g mushrooms

3 shallots

1 bouquet garni

10 cl. White wine

30 cl. Veal stock

20 cl. Of fresh cream

1 bunch of tarragon

3 sprigs of parsley

1 tbsp. Flour

6 potatoes

20 g. Butter

1 tbsp. Tablespoons

Salt and pepper from the mill

Preparation

1.   Peel the shallots and chop them. Cut the mushrooms in four.

2.   Cut the chicken into eight pieces.

3.   Inside a casserole, dissolve the butter with the oil and fry the pieces of chicken. Add shallots and mushrooms and fry for 5 minutes.

4.   Add the flour, moisten with the white wine. Add the veal stock, the bouquet garni, and the potatoes. Season, cover and cook for 30 minutes. Finally, add the liquid cream and cook another 10 minutes.

5.   Serve with parsley and chopped tarragon on top.

Nutrition Facts

Serving Size: 1 serving

Amount per Serving

Calories   606.4

Total Fat 44.6 g

Total Carbohydrate   1.5 g

Dietary Fiber   0.0 g

Sugars   0.0 g

Protein   48.4 g

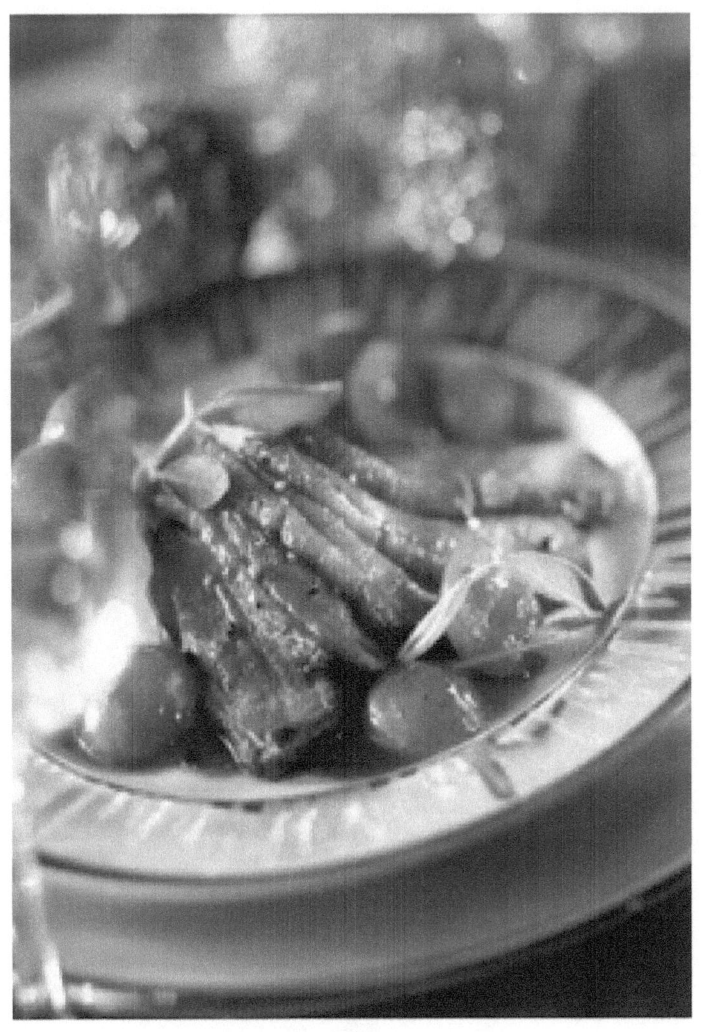

For: 4 people

Preparation time: 15 minutes

Cooking time: 15 minutes

Ingredients

2 duck breast (or fillet) approximately 350 g each

300 g frozen Mirabelle plums (or fresh)

1 tsp. chicken, ground coffee

3 cl of plum brandy

50 g of cold butter

Salt and pepper from the mill

Preparation

1. Let the Mirabelle thaw at room temperature.
2. Remove some fat from the sides of the breasts. Cut the skin in crosspieces, using a sharp knife. Put them skin side in a hot pan, without adding fat. Cook for 6 minutes on high heat. Turn them over and simmer for 4 minutes. Let them rest on a plate covered with aluminum foil.
3. Empty the grease from the pan without wiping it. Throw in Mirabelle plums and cook for 2 to 3 minutes while stirring. Remove them from the frying pan and retain them warm. Replace with the bottom of poultry diluted in water and the brandy. Bring to the boil by peeling off the cooking juices with a wooden spoon. Stir in small pieces of butter while whisking.
4. Slice the duck breasts. Stir the juice in the sauce. Mix.
5. Arrange the slices of filleted duck on the plates, Pour the sauce and add the mirabelles. Serve immediately.

Nutrition Facts

Calories 102   (427 kJ)

Calories from fat 32

% Daily Value 1

Total Fat 3.5g 5%

Sat. Fat 1.1g   5%

Protein   16.5g

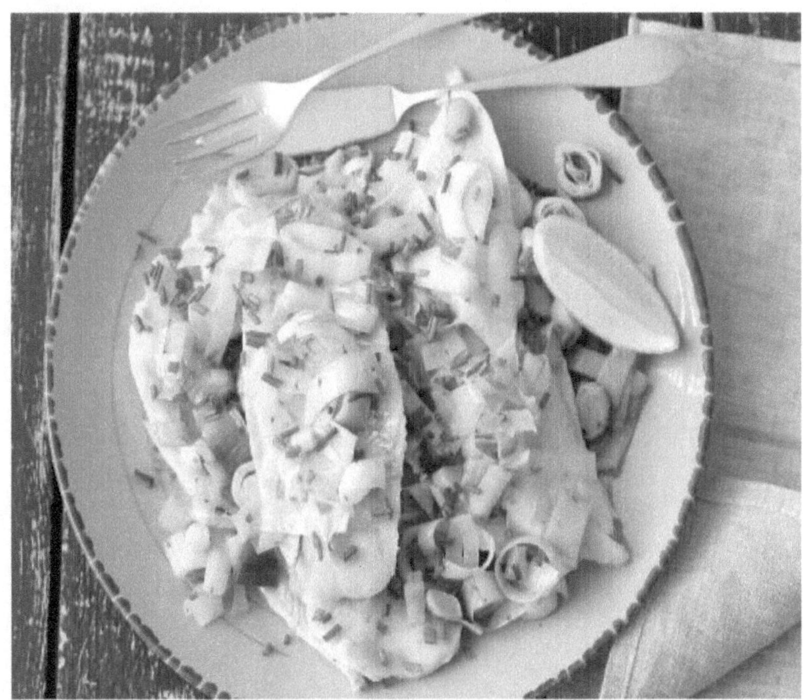

5. Steamed Cod

For 4 portions

Preparation: 30 min

The high-quality protein in the cod stimulates the metabolism and serves as a building material for cells, muscles, enzymes, and hormones. Valuable proteins also prevent cravings and muscle breakdown.

Ingredients

Four cod fillets (à 150 g)

4 tbsps. Lemon juice

2 bars leek

3 tbsps. Rapeseed oil

100 ml of vegetable stock

Salt

Pepper

½ dried thyme

½ bunch chives (10 g)

One organic lemon

Preparation

1. Rinse the fish fillets, pat dry and drizzle with 2 tbsps. lemon juice. Clean leeks, wash and cut into rings.
2. Heat 1 tbsps. Oil in a pan, dab fish dry, sauté for 2 minutes at medium heat. Then turn over, add the remaining lemon juice and 50 ml of vegetable stock and cover, cook for 5-7 minutes on low heat.
3. Meanwhile, heat remaining oil in a saucepan, sauté the leek rings in medium heat for 2 minutes, season with salt, pepper, and thyme. Add remaining vegetable stock and cook the leek for 5 minutes over low heat.
4. Meanwhile, wash chives, shake dry and cut into small rolls. Rinse lemon hot and cut into quarters
5. Season fish fillets and leeks with salt and pepper, arrange on plates and garnish with chives and lemon quarters.

<u>Nutritional Fact</u>

Calories: 226 kcal

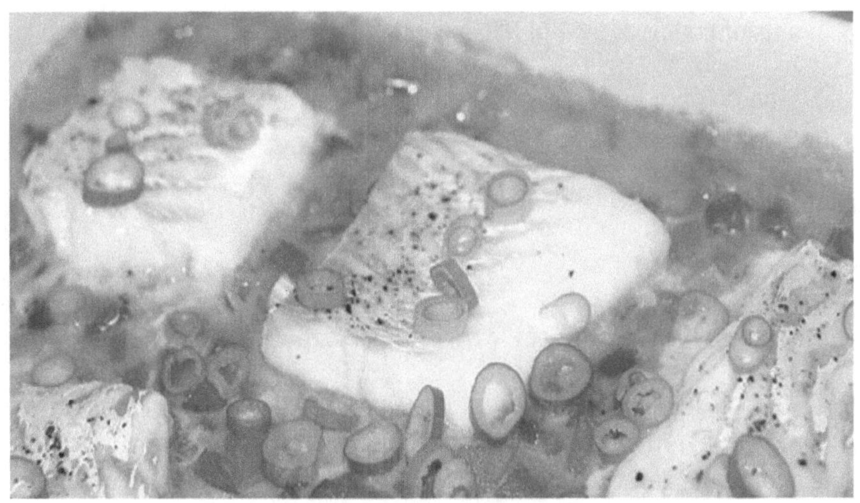

6. Fish in Bowl with Coconut Milk

Really simple recipe for fish and vegetables in dishes with a creamy coconut milk sauce, mild red curry and a hint of lime

For 4 people

Ingredients

400 grams of carrots

2 tablespoons of oil

2 teaspoons of red curry paste (or "regular curry" to taste)

1 clove of garlic

4 peppers

1 ds of coconut milk

Juice from 1 lime fruit

Salt

Pepper

600 grams of cod or other white fish

1 tablespoon of cornstarch or wheat flour for smoothing (can be easily omitted)

1 night spring onion

Preparation

1. Peel and cut the carrots. Set the oven to 200 degrees.

2. Put the oil in the pan and wipe the curry paste (or normal curry) over medium heat. Put the carrots in the pan and let them cook for a few minutes while cutting the garlic and peppers. Stir in the carrots, so they do not burn.

3. Cut the garlic, cut into thin slices and place on the pan. Rinse the peppers, cut into cubes and place in the pan. Take a few minutes to allow the peppers to add some liquid, and small bites begin to soften.

4. Add the coconut milk and cook over low heat. Try the coconut sauce with lime juice, salt, and pepper. Even if necessary, stir the sauce with cornmeal or wheat flour in a little cold water.

5. Clean the spring onions, cut into slices and mix in the sauce (leave something to sprinkle the finished bowl).

6. Clean the fish and dip it dry with a small paper towel or a clean dishcloth, Season with salt and pepper.

7. Pour the coconut sauce into a pan and place the pieces of fish on top. Stir the oven for about 12 minutes or until the fish is tender but still juicy.

8. Sprinkle the last spring onions over it and eat the shell as it is.

Nutritional Fact

270kcal per 100g

39.2g

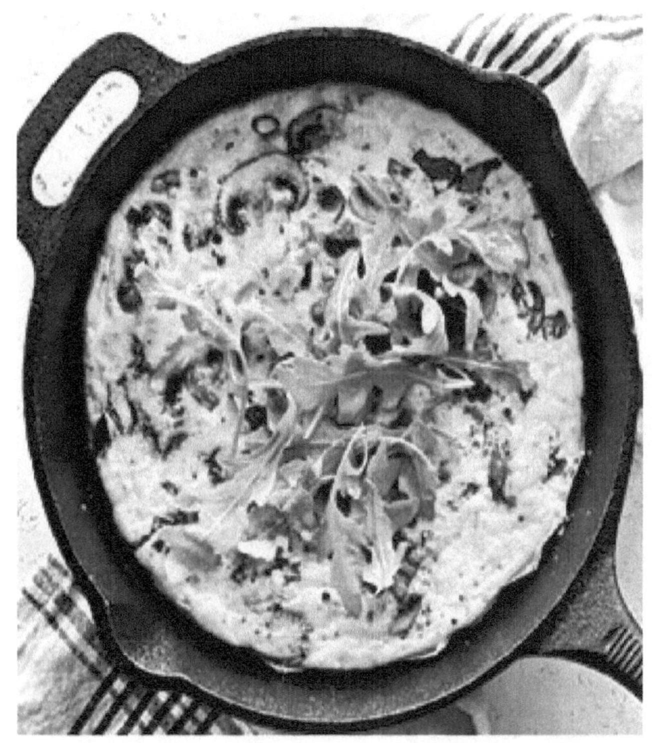

7. Ketogenic Frittata of Goat Cheese and Mushrooms

Prep time: 30 mins

2 portions

Ingredients

Frittata

150 g mushrooms

75 g fresh spinach

50 g chives

50 g butter

6 eggs

110 g goat cheese

Salt and ground black pepper

At your service

150 g green leafy vegetables

2 tbsp olive oil

Salt and ground black pepper

Preparation

1. Preheat the oven temperature to 175 ° C (350 ° F).
2. Grate or crumble the cheese and mix in a bowl with the eggs. Salt and pepper to taste.
3. Cut the mushrooms into small pieces. Chop the chives.
4. Dissolve the butter over medium heat in a pan suitable for the oven and fry the mushrooms and onions for 5-10 minutes or until golden brown.
5. Add the spinach to the pan and fry for another 1-2 minutes. Pepper.
6. Pour the egg mixture in the pan. Bake it for 20 minutes or till browned and firm in the middle.
7. Serve with green leafy vegetables and olive oil.

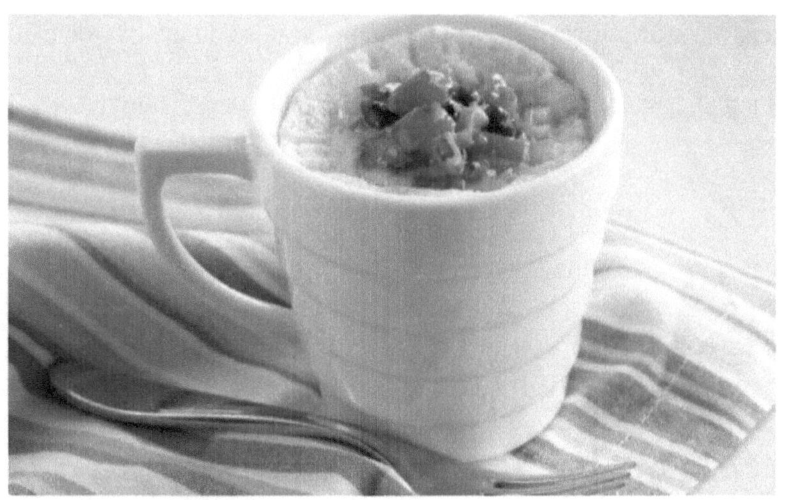

8. Scrambled eggs in a cup

Prep time: 3 mins

1 portion

Ingredients

2 eggs

2 tbsp cream to beat

Salt and pepper

1 tbsp butter

Preparation

1.   Grease a large cup or bowl with mild butter. Beat the eggs and the cream to beat. Fill the cup to a maximum of two thirds, as the eggs will gain volume when cooked.

2.   Add a pinch of salt including freshly ground black pepper or cayenne.

3.   Cook into the microwave at maximum power for 1-2 minutes (700 watts). Stir and microwave another minute. Have in mind that the eggs are

however made after removing them from the heat, so do not overdo them.

4.   Remove and add a little butter. Allow cooling for one minute.

Nutrition

Ketogenic low in carbons

Per portion

Net carbohydrates: 2% (1 g)

Fiber: 0 g

Fat: 84% (31 g)

Protein: 15% (12 g)

kcal: 329

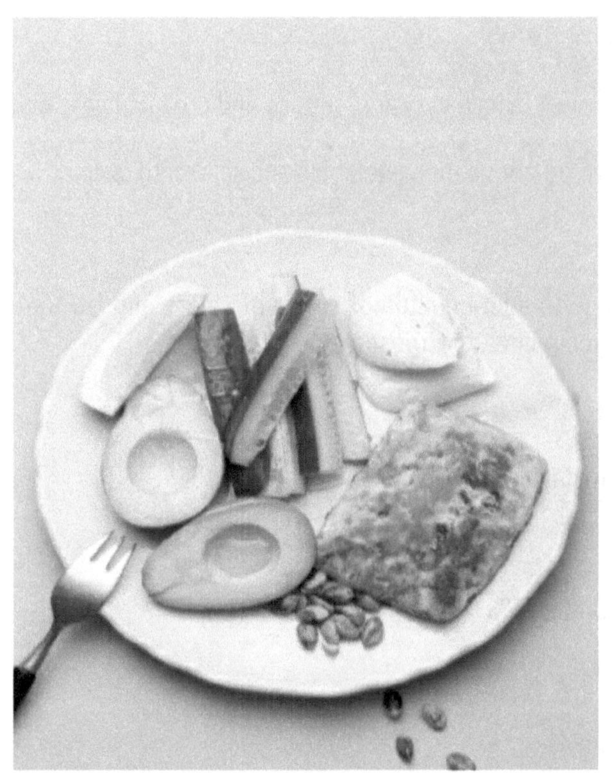

9. Keto plate of turkey

Prep time: 5 mins

2 portions

Ingredients

175 g turkey cold cuts

2 avocados

75 g (75 ml) cream cheese

50 g lettuce

60 ml of olive oil

Salt or pepper

Preparation

1. Put the turkey, sliced avocado, lettuce and cream cheese on a plate.

2. Pour olive oil above the vegetables and season to taste.

Advice!

Do not hesitate to add a couple of sticks of celery and fill the hollow of the celery with cream cheese. Crocante!

Nutrition Facts

Ketogenic low in carbons

Per portion

Net carbohydrates: 4% (9 g)

Fiber: 14 g

Fat: 84% (75 g)

Protein: 12% (24 g)

Kcal: 820

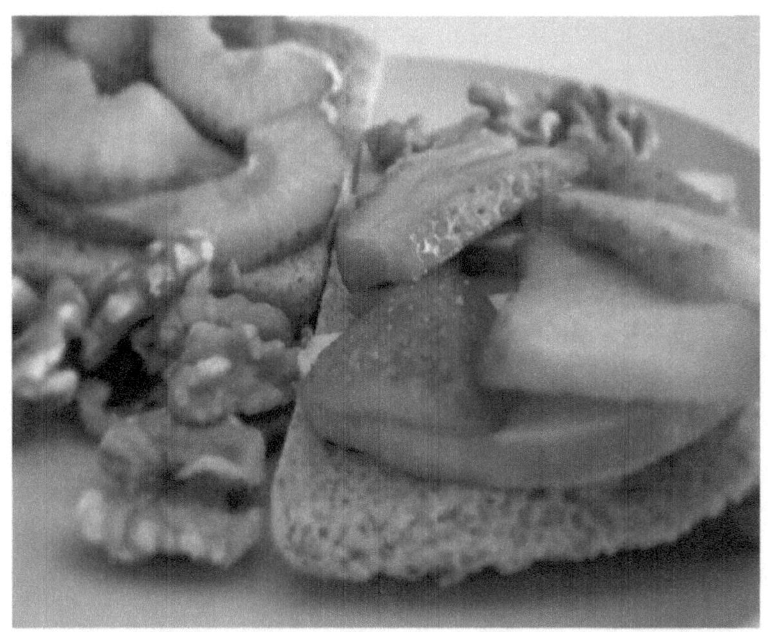

10. **Toast with Avocado and Strawberry Snack For Breakfast**

1 serving

Ingredients

2 slices wholemeal bread

1/2 avocado

2 strawberries

Extra virgin olive oil

1 pinch salt

Accompanying nuts

Preparation

1. Put the bread to toast and while you prepare the strawberries and avocado
2. Peel the avocado and make slices
3. Peel the tail of the strawberry, wash it well and make slices
4. Put olive oil on the bread, on avocado, on strawberries, a little salt and oil and ... enjoy! And with some nuts, it's already perfect!

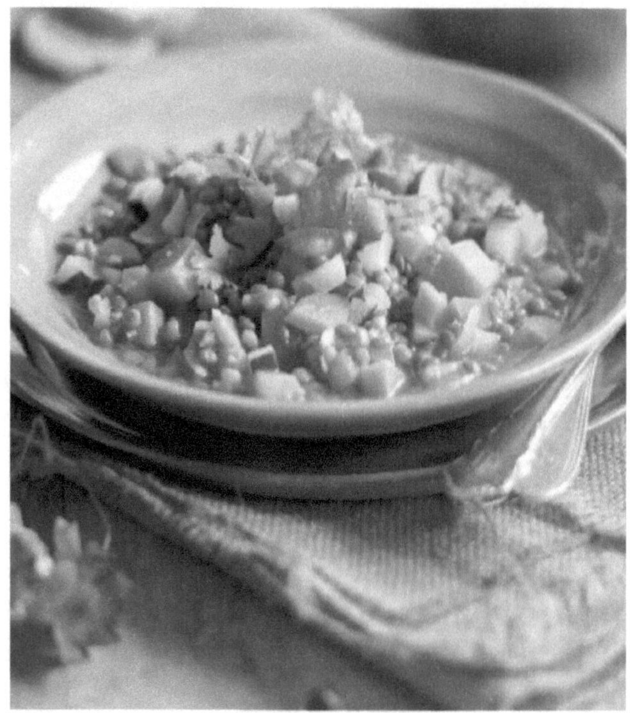

11. Light Lentil Stew

Ingredients:

250 g of brownish lentils

One zucchini

Two carrots

One onion

One clove garlic

One bay leaf

Two small branch tomatoes

One piece of ginger (optional)

Three teaspoons of olive oil

Two sprigs of coriander or parsley

Salt and pepper

Preparation

1. Prepare the vegetables. First, peel the onion and the garlic, and chop them. Then, peel the ginger, and chop it too fine. And finally, peel the carrot, wash the zucchini, remove them, and cut them into cubes.
2. Sauté the vegetables. Heat 2 teaspoons of oil in a casserole, add half of the onion and garlic and cook for approximately 4 minutes or so. Then add the ginger, bay leaf, carrot, and zucchini, and sauté a little.
3. Cook the lentils. After sautéing the vegetables, add the lentils. Cover with 3/4 of a litre (750 ml) of water, and cook over low heat for 45 minutes till the lentils are tender, and reserve.
4. Assemble the plate.
5. Finally, wash the tomatoes and chop them. Mix them with the rest of the onion and garlic, and season them with salt, pepper and the remaining oil. Divide the lentils into four bowls or bowls, and add the tomato hash and some leaves of coriander or parsley.
6. And if you want a fresh and ultra-fast version, instead of stewing the lentils, you can buy them already cooked and make a salad. You have to sauté the vegetables a little, but not too much so that they remain al dente. And mix them with the lentils already cooked and drained, and the tomato

hash.

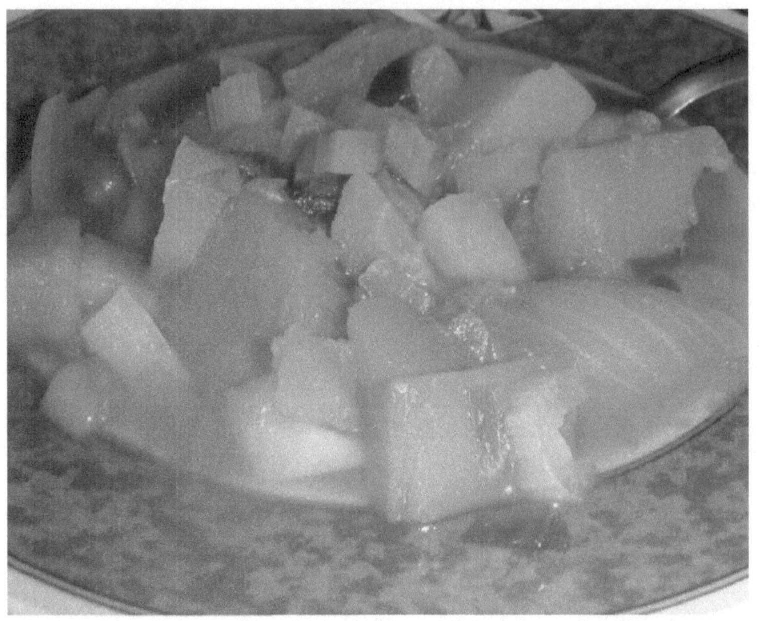

12. **Vegetable soup in an electric pressure cooker**

Ingredients

Six servings

Two green onions

Two leeks

Two celery sticks

Two carrots

One onion

Four slices pumpkin squash

Two medium potatoes

One zucchini round

Two cubes vegetable broth

1 liter (200cc) water

Preparation

1. Cut celery, green and port and add to the pot.
2. Add the carrot and onion in 4 (in case someone prefers to remove it from the plate.) In my house, one of my children does not like it, and I leave it visible.
3. Then add the zucchini, pumpkin, and cubes of broth.
4. Finally the potato and cover with water.
5. Cover the pot and program. In this case soup. Traditionally, cook on low heat for about 1 hour since it boils.
6. Serve very warm, If you prefer to add noodles or a little rice.

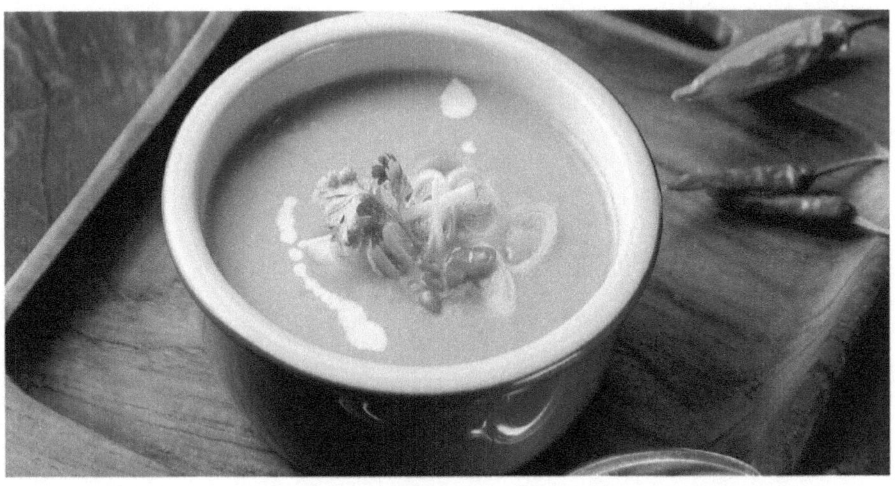

13.　　　Thai Pumpkin Soup

Creamy pumpkin soup with a hint of Thailand: coconut milk, ginger, and chili.

Ingredients

3EL Coconut Oil

500G Pumpkin

400G Carrots

1piece Spring Onion (50 G)

1piece Small Chili

1piece Clove Of Garlic

5cm Ginger (30 G)

1TL Turmeric

500ml Vegetable Stock

400ml Coconut Milk

5leaves Thai Basil

1piece Lime Leaf

Prize Salt

EL Soy Sauce

Heap Spoon Of Coconut Oil

Prize Black Pepper

1EL Lime Juice

Fresh coriander to serve

Preparation

1. Cut off the pumpkin drink. Peel pumpkin as needed hollow out the pumpkin and weigh it. Use the same amount of carrots. Peel carrots. Cut pumpkin and carrots into large

pieces. Peel ginger and turmeric. Finely chop the spring onion, chili, ginger, turmeric, and garlic.

2. Heat coconut oil in a saucepan. Fry spring onion, ginger, chili, turmeric, and garlic. Add carrots and pumpkin and roast without browning. Add soup and coconut milk, add basil and lime leaf. Bring to a boil, add basil and lime leaf. Simmer on a flame for about 15 minutes until the vegetables are tender. Prick vegetables with a needle. If the vegetables slip off easily, it is soft.
3. Remove lime leaf and basil. Puree the soup with a hand blender.
4. Cook the lentils. After sautéing the vegetables, add the lentils. Cover with 3/4 of a litre (750 ml) of water, and cook over low heat for 45 minutes till the lentils are tender, and reserve.

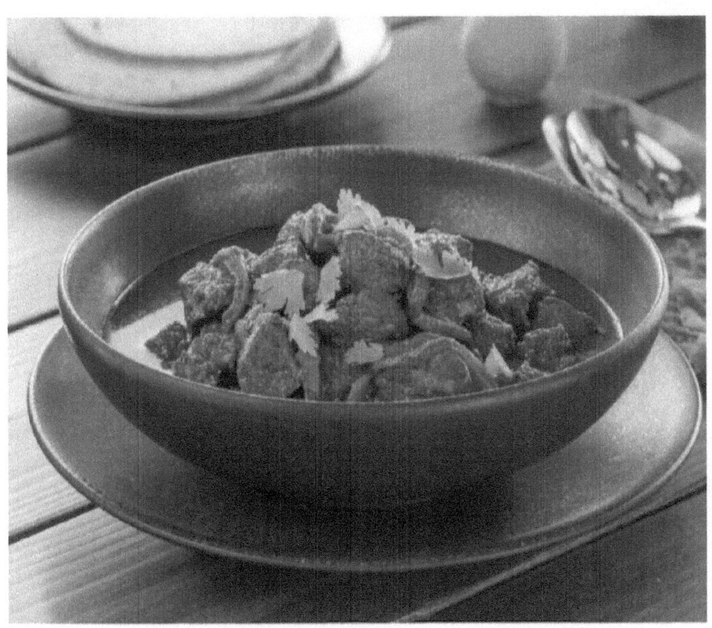

14.   Meat stew with nopales

Weather: 30 min. Approx.

Servings: 5 approx.

Ingredients

1 kilo of beef skirt

6 clean and chopped nopales

3 tomatoes

1 onion

1/2 sweet pepper

2 cloves of garlic

Oil

Salt and pepper

1 pinch of baking

Preparation

1. Cook the beef skirt in a pressure cooker for 45 minutes, with a pinch of salt. Save the meat broth.

2. Discard the meat and fry lightly, together with the sliced onion, tomato, chili, and garlic.

3. Cook apart the nopales with a little salt and a pinch of bicarbonate.

4. Drain cooked nopales and wash.

5. Pour the nopales into the meat fry with the rest of the ingredients.

6. Add a little stock of meat and let cook for 15 minutes.

Nutritional Information

Calories   107.3

Total Fat   0.9 g

Total Carbohydrate   24.2 g

Dietary Fiber   6.0 g

Sugars   0.0 g

Protein   4.2 g

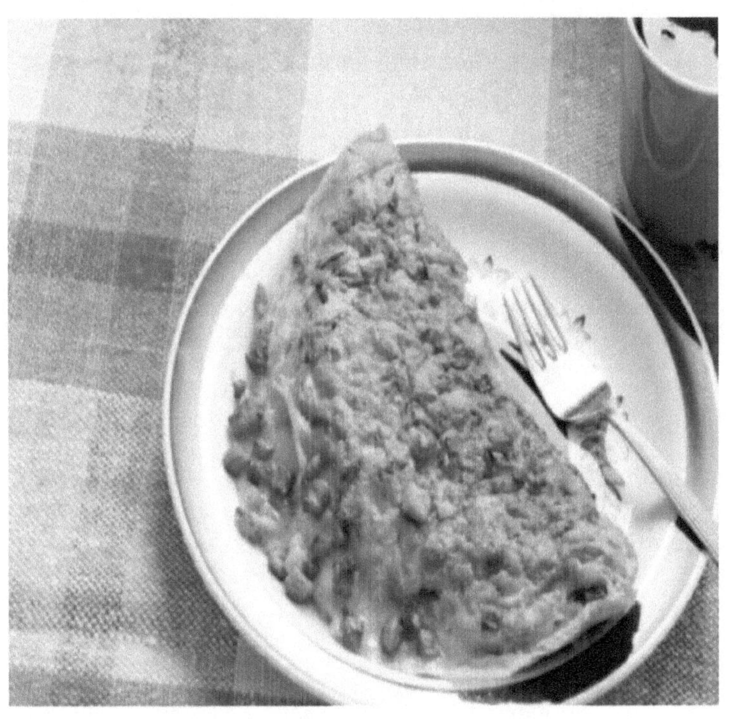

15.   Omelet of Keto Cheese

Prep time: 15 mins

2 portions

Ingredients

75 g butter

6 eggs

200 g shredded cheddar cheese

Salt and black pepper ground to taste

Preparation

1. Beat the eggs until soft and lightly frothy. Add half of the blended cheddar cheese and mix. Salt and pepper to taste.
2. Melt the butter in a hot pan. Pour the egg mixture and let stand for a few minutes.
3. Lower the heat and continue cooking until the egg mixture is almost done. Add the remaining grated cheese. Fold and serve immediately.

Advice!

Flavor your creation with herbs, chopped vegetables or even Mexican sauce. And do not hesitate to cook the tortilla with olive oil or coconut oil to have a different flavor profile.

Nutrition Facts

Ketogenic low in carbons

Per portion

Net carbohydrates: 2% (4 g)

Fiber: 0 g

Fat: 81% (80 g)

Protein: 18% (40 g)

kcal: 897

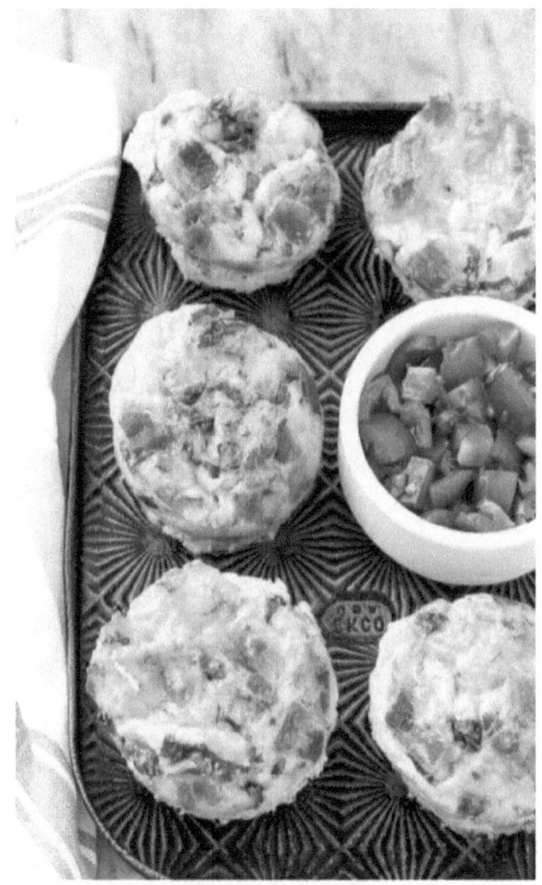

16.   Egg muffins

Prep time: 25 mins

4 portions

Ingredients

8 eggs

1 spring onion, finely chopped

150 g dried chorizo with air or salami or cooked bacon

75 g grated cheese

1 tbsp red pesto or green pesto (optional)

Salt and ground black pepper

Preparation

1. Preheat the oven temperature to 175 ° C (350 ° F).
2. Chop the chives and meat finely.
3. Beat the eggs together with the condiments and the pesto. Add the cheese and mix.
4. Put the dough into muffin molds and add bacon, sausage or salami.
5. Bake it for approximately 25 minutes, depending on the size of the mold.

Tips!

Kids love these muffins full of cheese. They are perfect for carrying in the lunch box.

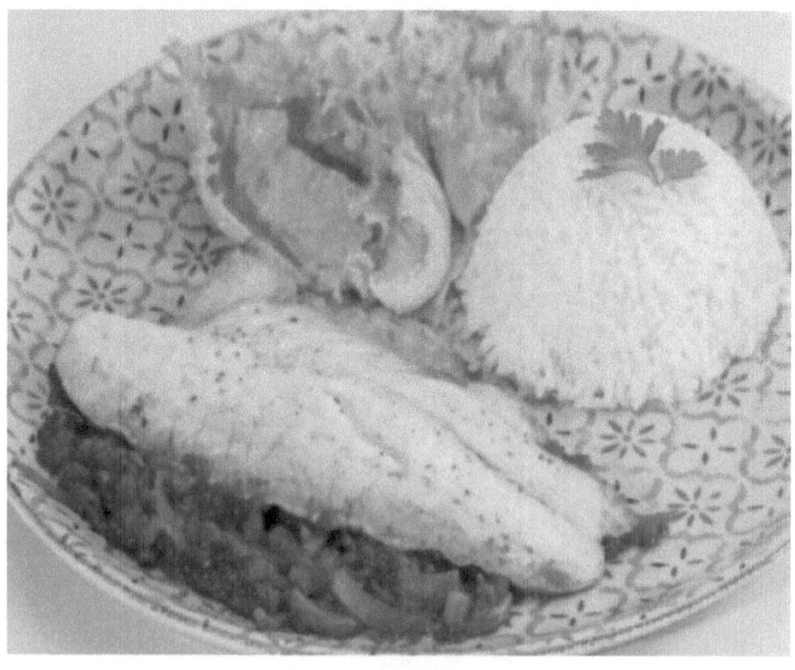

17.   Fish Sauce Peppers

For 3 people:

Ingredients

3 fish fillets

1 can (300g) of peppers in oil

2 tbsp. coffee sugar

4 tbsp. soy sauce

2 tbsp. maizéna

1 small red pepper

1Cuil. Ginger soup

Salt and pepper

Preparation

1. Season the fish and sprinkle with ginger.

2. Drain the peppers. Mince the chili.

3. Mix the ingredients of the sauce, sugar, soy sauce, maizena and 25cl of water.

4. Sear the fish in a drizzle of oil, remove. Pour the sauce, chili and peppers, allow thickening. Serve with fish

Nutritional Fact

Cholesterol 109mg   36%

Sodium 86mg   4%

Potassium 967.12mg   28%

Carbohydrates 0g   0%

Dietary Fiber 0g   0%

Sugars 0g

Protein 39.2g

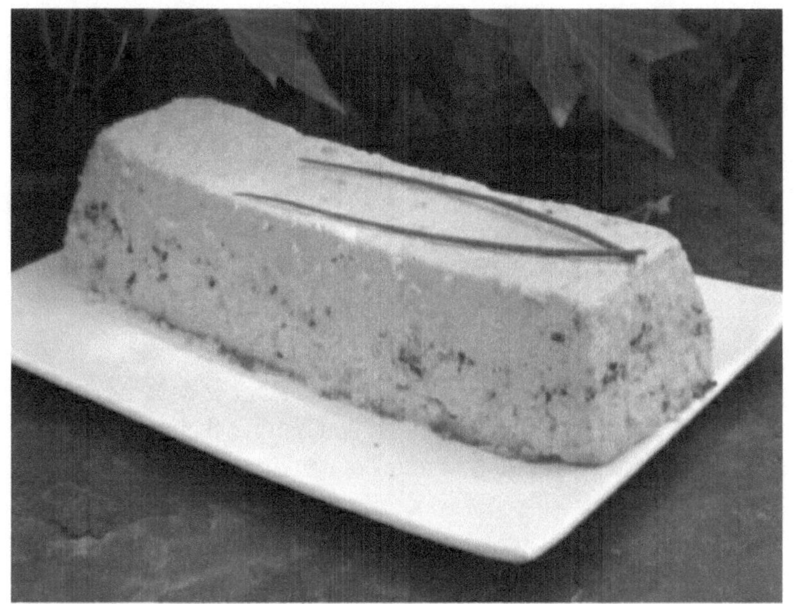

30 minutes

Ingredients

1 bar

300 g tomato coulis

1 tablespoon of olive oil

1 onion

1/2 cc of turmeric

1/2 cc of cumin

1/2 cc of garam masala

Salt and pepper

1 small piece of fresh ginger

1 bowl of rice

Preparation

1. Peel the onion and slice it.
2. Grate the ginger.
3. Fry the onion with a little oil in the pan for 5 minutes.
4. Add the mixed spices.
5. Prolong cooking for a few minutes.
6. Add the coulis and cook for 10 minutes covered.
7. Meanwhile, raise the fillets of bar if you have not asked your fishmonger to do it and remove their skin.
8. Add them for 5 minutes of cooking. Add salt and pepper.
9. Serve with cooked rice (a volume of rice for a volume and a half of water with a pinch of salt).

Nutritional Fact

Cholesterol 109mg   36%

Sodium 86mg   4%

Potassium 967.12mg   28%

Carbohydrates 0g   0%

Dietary Fiber 0g   0%

Sugars 0g

Protein 39.2g

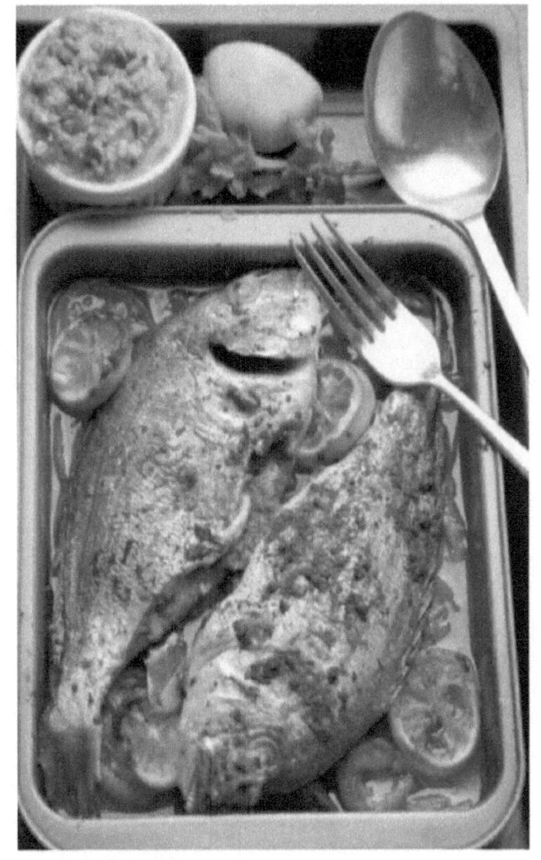

| 19. | Baked Sea Bream in Lebanese Style |

Ingredients:

For the dish:

1 kilogram of whole fish type bream, salmon or trout

1 teaspoon of salt

1 teaspoon of cumin

1 teaspoon sweet pepper (paprikas)

1 onion

1 lemon

2 bay leaves

3 tomatoes

For the sauce:

3 cloves of garlic

1 tablespoon coriander seeds

1/2 teaspoon of salt

100 g of onion

1/2 bunch of green coriander

65 g of tahini (sesame puree)

1 lemon or about 50 ml of lemon juice

1/2 glass of vegetable oil (sunflower or olive)

10 g pine nuts

25 g chopped walnuts

1/2 to 1 teaspoon of fine cayenne pepper powder (according to taste)

1 pinch of pepper

Preparation:

1. Wash the fish; rub both sides with a teaspoon of salt, sweet pepper, and cumin. Inside a large baking tray, add the onion, tomatoes, and lemon sliced and put the fish and bay leaf. Add 1 glass of water. Sprinkle with a drizzle of olive oil.

2. Heat the oven temperature to 180 ° C. Put the tray in the oven and cook for 20 minutes or 25 minutes depending on the type and thickness of the fish.

3. With a pestle, crush garlic, salt, and coriander seeds until coriander becomes powder. Set aside.

4. Minute an onion, finely chop green coriander and leave aside.

5. In a large bowl, pour tahini, lemon juice, and 100 ml water, mix well until you obtain a homogeneous liquid, then reserve.

6. In a saucepan, add vegetable oil, heat over medium heat. Brown the pine nuts drain them.

7. In the same saucepan and remaining oil, brown the chopped onion. Add green coriander, the garlic-cilantro mixture in seeds and chopped walnuts and pepper. Simmer another 10 minutes. Finally, add tahini, lemon, and water. Cook for about 10 minutes. 8. Add the chili, mix and remove from the heat. Leave this sauce aside for dressing.

To serve, place the fish on a large plate, decorate with slices of peppers, tomatoes or any other vegetable to give color. Put the sauce on the fish, and then scatter over the pine nuts.

Good realization and good tasting!

Nutritional Fact

Potassium 967.12mg   28%

Carbohydrates 0g   0%

Dietary Fiber 0g   0%

Sugars 0g

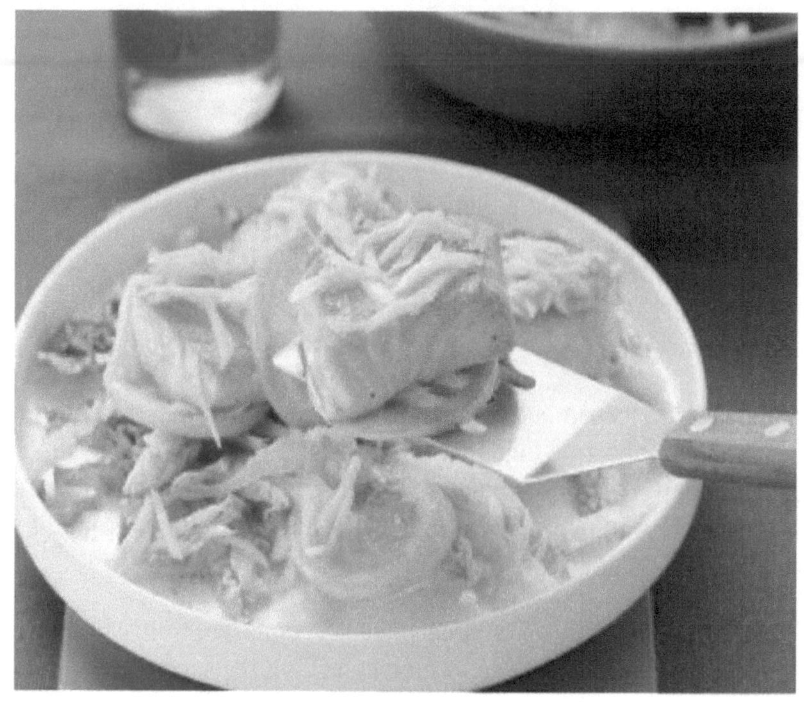

20.   Salmon with lemon and ginger

Preparation: 20 min

Calories: 338 kcal

Even if there are lower-fat fish, the salmon is fit for a diet especially in combination with lemon and lettuce hearts. By the way: The omega-3 fatty acids in salmon can even boost fat loss in the body.

For 4 portions

Ingredients

2 romaine lettuce hearts

600 g salmon fillet

1 piece ginger (20 g)

2 organic lemons

Salt

Pepper

2 tbsps. olive oil

75 ml of vegetable stock

1 tsp. honey

Preparation

1. Wash lettuce hearts, spin dry, cut into strips and spread on 4 plates.
2. Rinse salmon fillet under cold water, pat dry and cut into coarse pieces. Peel ginger and cut into fine pens. 1 lemon hot wash, pat dry and slice halve the rest of the lemon and squeeze out the juice.
3. Season salmon with salt and pepper. Melt the oil in a pan and fry the salmon with ginger and lemon slices in medium heat until golden brown in 3-4 minutes. Remove salmon pieces from the pan. Serve with ginger and lemon on the salad.
4. Deglaze the stock with broth and lemon juice. Season with honey, salt, and pepper and drizzle the salad with it.

Nutritional Fact

Protein   31 g   (32%)

Fat   22 g   (19%)

Carbohydrates   3 g   (2%)

Added sugar   1 g   (4%)

Roughage   1 g   (3%)

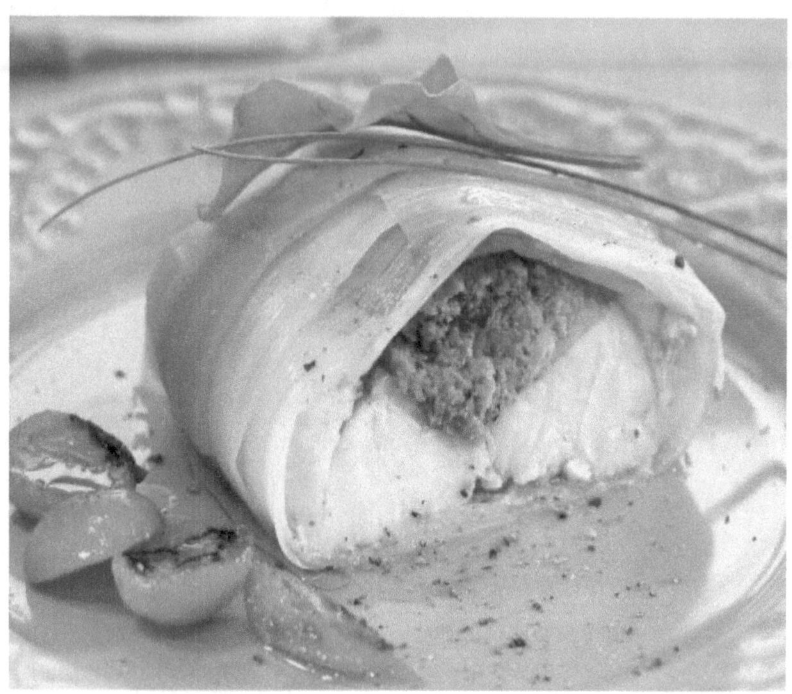

21.   Monkfish and spinach parcels

Time preparation: 45 minutes

The sea fish provides plenty of iodine and protein. Both ensure a smooth flow of metabolism. The spicy-tasting leek is very rich in zinc and thus has a wound-healing an immune-boosting effect.

For 4 portions

Ingredients

50 g spinach

Salt

2 bars leek

Two big carrots (300 g)

600 g monkfish

One organic lemon

300 g seelachsfilet

100 ml of soy cream

150 g cottage cheese (0.3% fat)

Pepper

100 ml fish stock (glass)

250 g yellow or red cherry tomatoes

1 tbsp. olive oil

Four red sorrel orchard leaves at will

¼ bunch chives (5 g)

Preparation

1.   Clean, wash, and drizzle the spinach in boiling salted water and let it collapse in 1-2 minutes. Remove spinach, chill cold, squeeze well, chop and chill.

2.   Clean the leeks cut in length and wash. Separate the leaves from each other and add to the boiling salted water for 2 minutes. Then remove cold quench and dab dry.

3.   Clean and peel the carrots, cut lengthways into thin strips, and add to the boiling salted water for 3 minutes until soft. Remove, chill off cold and dab carrot strips dry.

4.   Wash monkfish fillet and pat dry. Lay the bottom of an ovenproof mold slightly overlapping with the leek and carrot strips. Place the monkfish filet in the middle of it.

5.   Rinse the lemon hot, rub dry, rub the skin, and squeeze the juice. Cut the salmon filet into small pieces and puree with soy cream, cottage cheese and

spinach to a fine mass. Season the mixture with salt, pepper, lemon peel, and juice, spread on the fillet and beat the vegetable strips over the fish from both sides.

6.   Add seelachsfilet, fish stock and cook the monkfish fillet in a preheated oven at 180°C (160°C convection, gas: stage 2-3) for about 30 minutes.

7.   In the meantime wash and halve cherry tomatoes. In a frying pan, add olive oil fry the tomatoes in it for about 5 minutes over medium heat.

8.   Wash red sorrel orchard leaves and chives and shake dry. Cut monkfish fillet in leek and carrot clove into four pieces and arrange with tomatoes, lettuce leaves, and chives.

Nutritional Fact

Calories: 351 kcal

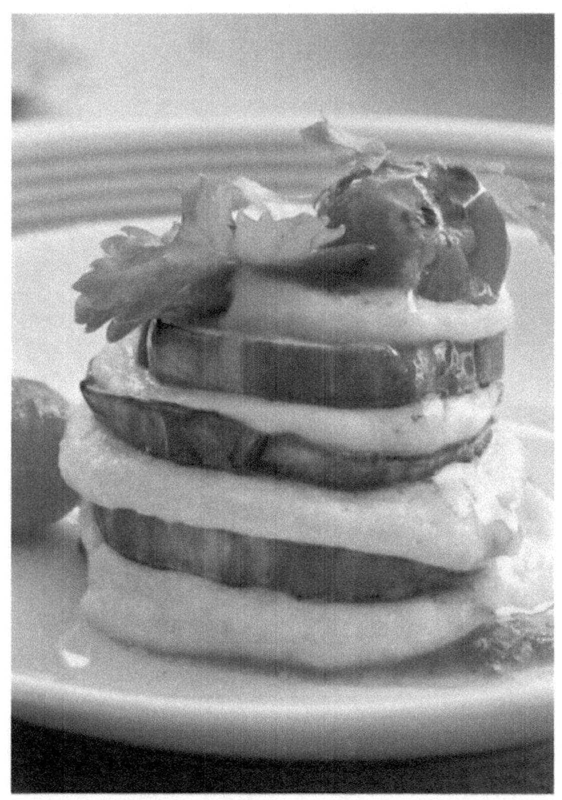

22.　　　Timbale of eggplant and hummus

A very healthy recipe based on chickpeas and aubergines to incorporate more legumes to the diet with a festive look.

Ingredients:

3 eggplants

300 g cooked chickpeas

1 clove garlic

1 lemon juice

1 tbsp. of tahini

8-12 cherry tomatoes

2 tbsps. extra virgin olive oil

1 tsp. ground cumin

A ½ cup of parsley leaves

Pepper

Salt

Preparation

1. Bake the eggplants, clean the aubergines and then cut them into slices about a ½ centimeter. Next, you spread a baking tray with oil and place the eggplant slices in it, sprinkle them, and roast at 180 ° C for about 15-20 minutes or so.
2. Make the hummus. To do this, wash the chickpeas and crush them with the peeled garlic, the lemon juice, the tahini, and the cumin. Then, salt and mix until there is dough with a fine texture. Then if necessary, add a little water. Do not miss our recipe for light hummus.
3. Prepare the accompaniment. On the one hand, blanch the parsley, refrigerate it and crush it with the oil. And then, on the other hand, brown the tomatoes and reserve.
4. Assemble the plate, sandwich eggplant slices with layers of hummus to form a milfoil type timbale. And it is accompanied with the golden tomatoes, a touch of parsley oil on top and the plate, and then use a few leaves of whole parsley.

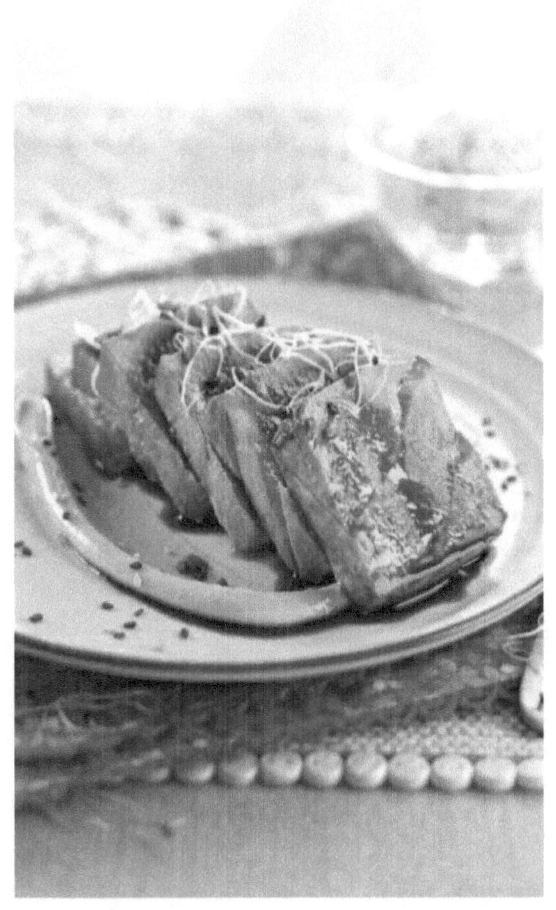

23.   Skewers of Tuna, Watermelon, and Avocado

Three ingredients that, separately, are very good and, together, are even more so. Prepare this delicious recipe by following a few simple steps.

Ingredients:

400 g of tuna loin

500 g of watermelon

1 lemon

1 dl of soy sauce

2 teaspoons of sesame seeds

2 avocados

2 teaspoons of sugar

2 sprigs of chives

Olive oil

Pepper and salt

Preparation

1. Clean and chop the fish and watermelon. On the one hand, wash the tuna and cut it into regular cubes. And on the other hand, clean and peel the watermelon. And cut 400 g into cubes of the same size as the tuna.
2. Reduce watermelon and soybeans. Tritura the 100 g of watermelon left over to obtain a juice. Strain this juice, put it in a saucepan on the fire with the sugar and the soy sauce, and reduce it by half with the soft fire and stirring. Season and let cool.
3. Assemble the skewers. Thread the tuna and watermelon cubes into each skewer, spread them with oil, sprinkle them and then leave it to marinate for 20 minutes or so.
4. Prepare the accompaniment. While the skewers are macerated, take advantage to peel the avocados quotes the bone and cut them into cubes. Add the lemon juice, 2 tablespoons of oil, the chives washed and chopped, salt, pepper and stir the mixture.
5. Grill the skewers and serve. Finally, broil the skewers on a plate greased with oil for 1 minute or so on each side. And once they are ready, spread the skewers with the soy and watermelon reduction, sprinkle with the sesame and serve them with the avocado as garnish

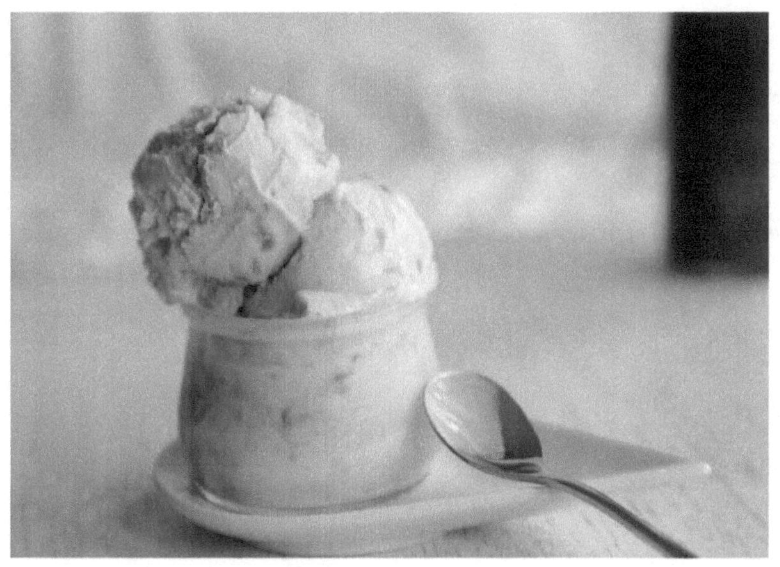

24.   Low carb strawberry with cheesecake ice cream and crunchy

Ingredients

For the cheesecake ice cream

200g cream cheese, double cream stage

200 l of cream

90ml of xylitol or erythritol

1 Msp. Ground vanilla

3 egg yolks

For the Strawberry Swirl

250ml strawberries frozen, fresh in summer

1/2 lemon (of which the juice)

40ml of xylitol or erythritol

For the meringue

3 egg whites

150 g of xylitol or erythritol

1/2 lemon (of which the juice)

Equipment

Ice cream machine

Piping bag

Nozzles

Preparation

1.   Freeze the ice bucket of your ice machine overnight (if you do not use a compressor machine).

2.   Weigh all ingredients and prepare — Thaw the strawberries.

3.   Mix the cream cheese with the cream and with the xylitol (amount for the cheesecake ice cream). Add the vanilla and heat the mixture on the stove. Stir well until the consistency is uniform and the cream cheese is dissolved.

4.   In a second pot, heat the thawed strawberries. Add the xylitol (for the Strawberry Swirl) and let the liquid simmer. Add the lemon juice.

5.   Allow both mixtures to cool in the refrigerator for at least 3 hours. When making ice cream, they must be cold (room temperature is not sufficient).

6.   Separate the eggs. Finely chop the xylitol (for the meringue) in a blender. Preheat the oven to 100 ° C (top/bottom heat). Cover the yolks and leave to cool.

7.   Beat the egg whites in a food processor with half of the powdery xylitol and the lemon juice very stiff. Slowly fold in the remaining powdery xylitol.

8.   Put the meringue inside a piping bag with the spout. Cover with a baking tray and with baking paper and sprinkle with it little meringue turrets. Let it dry on the bottom rail for 50 minutes (100 ° C top/bottom heat, if it gets too dark, put a baking tray over the meringue in the oven, if necessary reduce the temperature to 90 ° C and let it dry for up to 70 minutes). Then allow cooling.

9.   When the ice is well chilled, stir in the yolks. Insert the frozen container of the ice maker into the appliance. Fill the ice mass and start the stirrer.

10.   Puree the strawberry sauce (for fine fruit lines in the ice) or crush the strawberries roughly with the fork (for pieces of strawberry in the ice).

11.   If the low carb cheesecake ice cream is frozen in the machine, carefully fold in half of the fruit sauce. Crumble the cold meringues and fold in just as carefully.

12.   Keep the remaining fruit sauce and the remaining meringues for garnish.

13.   You can either enjoy the ice directly or freeze it. If you freeze the ice, you should let it thaw shortly before consumption, so you can easily scrape balls.

Nutrition Facts per ball (with erythritol, at 8 balls):

173.5 kcal

39.2 g carbohydrates

- Of which 4.1 g sugar (of course from dairy products and fruits)

- Of which 35 g sugar alcohols

- gives 4.2 g net carbohydrates 7.5 g protein 14.9 g fat

Nutrition facts per ball (with xylitol, at 8 balls):

275.5 kcal

39.2 g carbohydrates

- Of which 4.1 g sugar (naturally from dairy products and fruits)

- Of which 35 g sugar alcohols

7.5 g protein

14.9   g fat

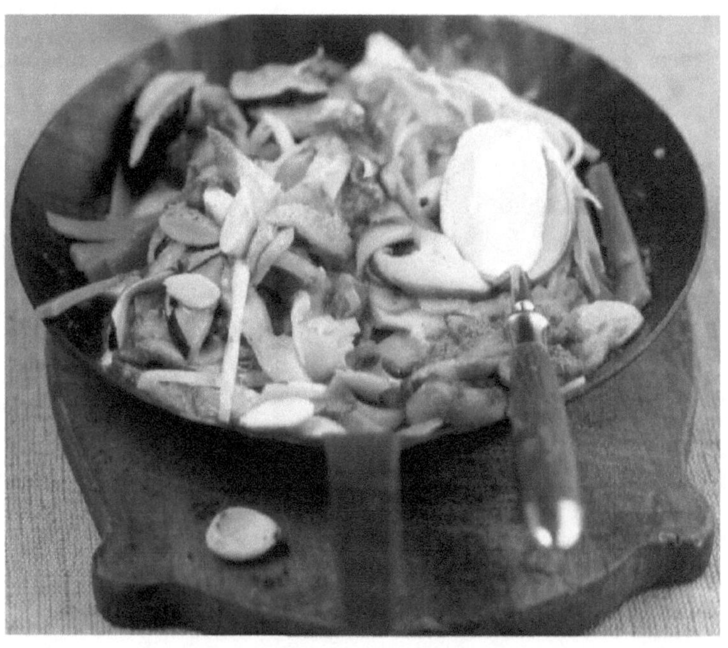

25.   Mushroom and vegetable pan with almonds

For 4 portions

Time preparation: 30 minutes

The colorful mixture of vegetables and mushrooms contains plenty of fiber, which ensures long-lasting satiety. Peppers also provide plenty of immunes boosting vitamin C; the carrots score with beta carotene, a precursor of vitamin A. The fat-soluble vitamin is essential for healthy eyes, among other things.

Ingredients

One big onion

Two garlic cloves

Three tomatoes

One red pepper

2 parsley

Two carrots

Salt

2 tbsps. Almonds (40 g)

400 g mixed mushrooms

1 tbsp. butter (15 g)

Pepper

1 splash Lemon juice

½ tbsp. Curry powder

2 tbsps. Sour cream (40 g)

Preparation

1. Peel onion and garlic and chop finely. Wash the tomatoes and slice into small cubes. Wash the pepper, clean and cut into thin strips.
2. Peel parsley roots and carrots, cut into thin sticks and blanch

in boiling salted water for 2 minutes. Drain, quench and drain.

3. Meanwhile roast almonds in a pan over medium heat without fat until they smell.
4. Clean and slice mushrooms. Heat the butter in a pan. Fry the onion and garlic over at medium heat until glassy. Add the pepper and simmer for 3 minutes.
5. Add mushrooms and simmer for 3-4 minutes over medium heat until they are ready. Add tomatoes, carrots and parsley roots and simmer for another 2 minutes. Season with salt, pepper, one dash of lemon juice and curry powder.
6. Add mushrooms and simmer for 3-4 minutes over medium heat until they are ready. Add tomatoes, carrots and parsley roots and simmer for another 2 minutes. Season with salt, pepper, one dash of lemon juice and curry powder.
7. Stir in sour cream and sprinkle with almonds.

Nutritional Fact

Calories: 203 kcal

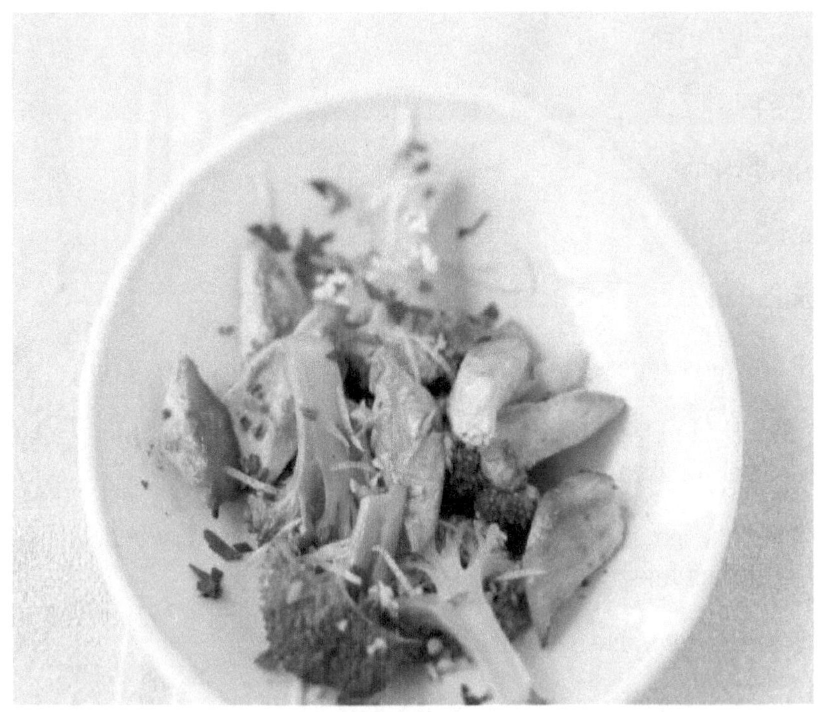

26.   Turkey strips with broccoli and lemon sauce

For 4 portions

Time preparation: 20 minutes

The tender poultry contains a lot of protein, which is essential for muscle building. Broccoli contains plenty of vitamins C. In addition to the chicken; the parsley contains considerable amounts of iron, which is necessary for the blood formation, among other things.

Ingredients

600 g turkey breast

800 g broccoli

Salt

One organic lemon

Two garlic cloves

3 stems parsley

2 tbsps. Sesame oil

Pepper

Preparation

1. Rinse turkey breast under cold water, dab dry and cut into strips.

2. Wash and clean broccoli, cut into florets and cook in boiling, slightly salted water for about 5 minutes.

3. Rinse the lemon hot, dab dry, peel off the zest, and squeeze out the juice. Peel garlic and finely chop.

4. Wash parsley, shake dry and finely chop.

5. Heat sesame oil inside a frying pan and roast the turkey strips in it for 2-3 minutes till it shows golden brown, season with salt and pepper. Add the lemon juice and some water as needed and add broccoli, lemon zest, and garlic. Let it simmer, add the parsley and season to taste.

Nutritional Fact

Calories: 250 kcal

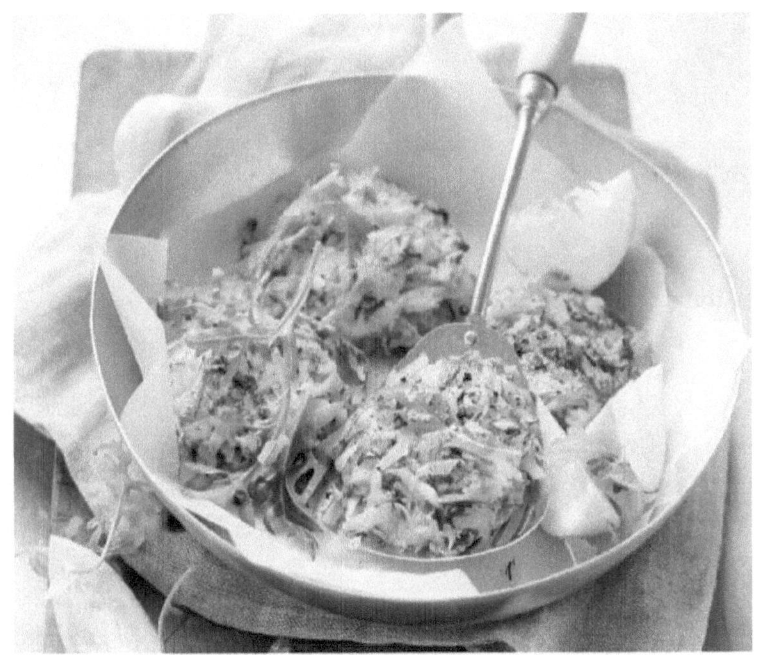

27.   Zucchini carrots buffer

For 4 portions

Time preparation: 30 minutes

Thanks to plenty of vegetables, these buffers contain a lot of fiber and make you full for a long time. Carrots contain a series of beta-carotene, a precursor of vitamin A. The fat-soluble vitamin is vital for healthy eyes.

Ingredients

500 g predominantly hard-boiling potatoes

Two carrots

One zucchini

1 tbsp. chickpea flour (15 g)

Salt

Nutmeg

2 tbsps. Olive oil

One organic lemon

½ bunch rocket (40 g)

Preparation

1. Peel potatoes. Wash carrots and zucchini and clean. Grate everything roughly and mix with the chickpea flour, season with salt and freshly grated nutmeg.
2. Heat olive oil inside a pan and add the potato mixture in portions. Press lightly flat and fry on medium heat from each side for about 6 minutes.

3. Meanwhile, wash the lemon hot, pat dry and cut into slices. Wash the rocket and spin dry. Arrange buffers on four plates and garnish with rocket. Lemon splits are enough.

Nutritional Fact

Calories: 167 kcal

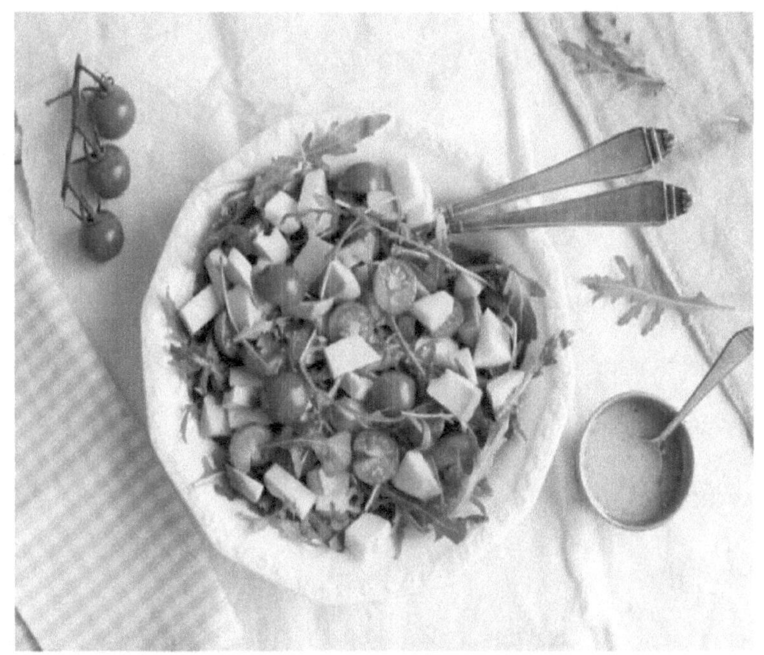

Time preparation: 15 minutes

Although avocados contain a lot of fat, because in addition to plenty of vitamin E score the green fruits with healthy polyunsaturated fatty acids, Mango has its yellow color due to the plant pigment beta carotene, which is a precursor of vitamin A, which is vital for healthy eyes. The cell-protecting lycopene from tomatoes completes the essential substance package.

Ingredients

For four portions

1 tbsp. lime juice

2 tbsps. White balsamic vinegar

2 tbsps. Rapeseed oil

2 tbsps. Olive oil

1 tsp. honey

1 tsp. medium hot mustard

Salt

Pepper

Three handful rocket (120 g)

200 g cherry tomatoes

One ripe mango

Two avocados

Preparation

1. For the vinaigrette, whip lime juice with balsamic vinegar, rapeseed and olive oils. Whisk in honey and mustard and then season with salt and pepper.
2. Wash the rocket and spin dry. Wash tomatoes and halve. Peel the mango, slice the pulp from the core and dice it. Halve the avocados, core them, remove the pulp from the skin and dice them as well. Add cherry tomatoes, ripe mango, avocados - all the salad ingredients inside a bowl with the vinaigrette and spread on four plates.

Nutritional Fact

Calories: 306 kcal

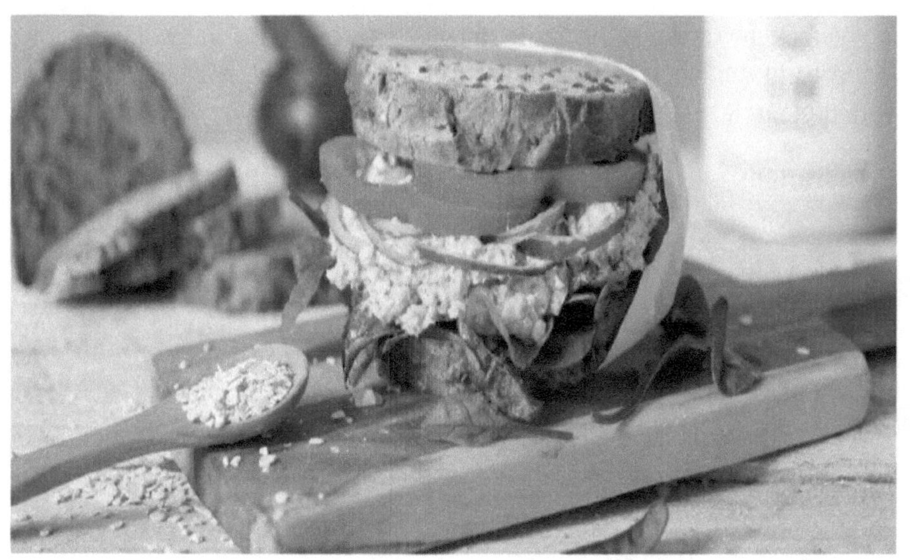

29.   Protein Sandwich with Tuna

Ideal for a busy day today

For 1 person

Ingredients: For tuna cream:

50 g   tuna in its juice

Two cts. Yogurt (1.5% fats)

1 tsp.   Mustard

1 tbsp.   Protein flakes Protein flakes

Salt, pepper, fresh parsley

For the bread:

Two slices

Protein bread Protein bread

Lettuce, pepper, onion rings

If you lack the time and the desire to cook but want to eat something healthy, this protein sandwich is made for you. It will be ready in a blink of an eye with protein flakes.

Preparation:

1. The sandwich of this recipe contains about 232 kcal and 33 g of protein.
2. Mix all the ingredients for the tuna cream in a small bowl and salt and pepper to taste.
3. Toast the slices of bread.
4. Place the lettuce leaves, tuna cream, pepper, and onion rings on one of the slices and close the sandwich with the other slice.
5. Then serve!!

Vegetarian variant

Replace the tuna with 50 g of canned chickpeas. Spread them with a fork and mix with the rest of the ingredients. It will be just as good as the sandwich in this recipe. Enjoy it also with spongy vegan protein pan.

Nutritional Facts:

Calories: 232

Carbohydrates: 6g

Protein: 33g

Fat: 6g

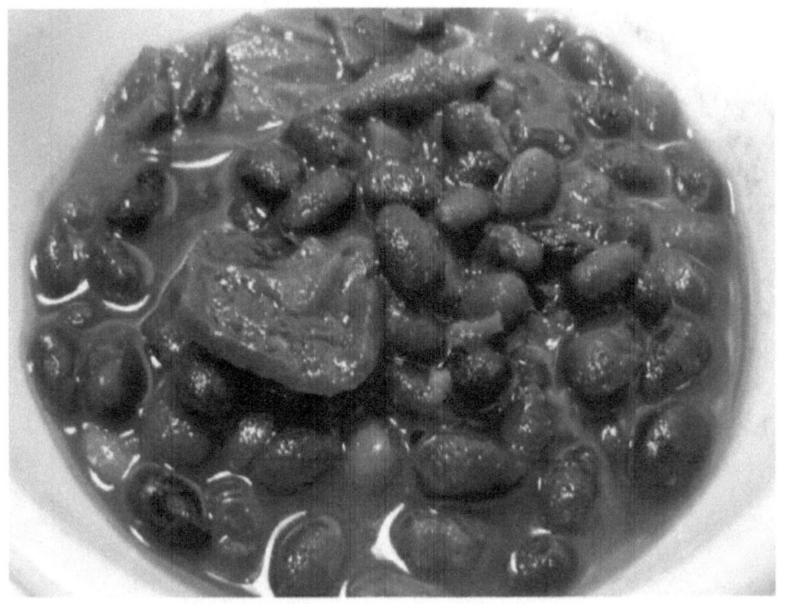

30. **Beans Charros Express**

In Jalisco, hot and dry can be made, and a ranchera sauce containing tomato, onion, and green chile is added. Also, in Mexico City, they are usually broths and are often eaten as soup.

Ingredients

1 kilo of bay beans

Five cloves of garlic

Six pieces of tomato without peel

One piece of onion

1/2 teaspoon of pepper

1/2 teaspoon ground cumin

250 grams of shredded Spanish chorizo

250 grams of smoked ham in cubes

250 grams of smoked bacon in cubes

250 grams of sausage

One sprig of finely chopped cilantro

100 grams of pork cracklings in chunks

Two chopped serrano chiles

To the taste of sea salt

Preparation

1. At night put to soak the beans, half onion, three garlic, and salt.
2. Boil the soaked beans, close the pressure pot Express and put the pressure regulator, place it in the stove with a high flame for about 25 minutes or until constant steam comes out, reduce the flame to the medium and cook for 1 hour.
3. Remove the Express Pressure Cooker from the heat, let cool, remove the pressure regulator, open the Express Pressure Cooker, and that's it!
4. Blend 3 tomatoes, half onion, two garlic, cumin, pepper, and reserve.
5. In a pan fry the chorizo sausage and the chef's suggestion. Accompany them with toast, avocado, and cheese. Bacon preparation, remove the fat that you release and add the sausages on casters, the diced ham, the chilies, and the three chopped tomatoes; already sautéed add the liquefied tomato sauce; once fried add the cooked beans and let boil over low heat.
6. To serve, put the cilantro and pork rind in pieces.

Presentation

Accompany them with toast, avocado, and cheese.

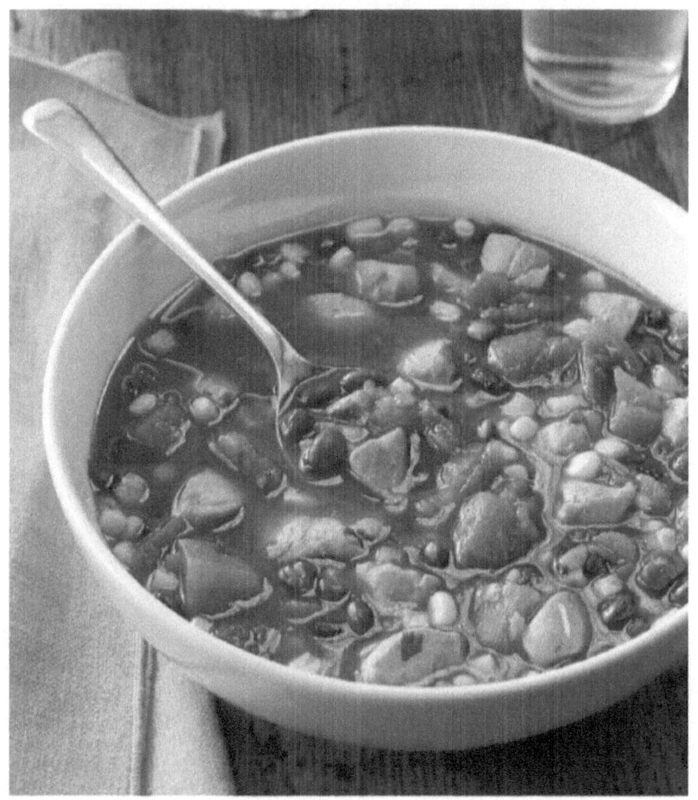

31. **Soup for slimming chicken and beans**

Serving portions: 8

Ingredients:

200 g of chicken breast

Salt

1 large chopped onion

1 teaspoon olive oil

2 cloves garlic, minced

2 cups chopped cherry tomatoes

2 chopped carrots

1 chopped green pepper

1 chopped pepper

1 tablespoon chili powder

1 ½ teaspoon cumin

½ tsp turmeric

½ teaspoon of paprika

¼ teaspoon dried oregano

4 cups low-sodium chicken broth

2 cups of corn

500 g of washed and drained black beans

¾ cup fresh coriander

1 cup of cheese

Preparation:

1. Cook the chicken breast in a pan filled with water over medium-high heat for 10 to 15 minutes;
2. After he's ready to shred it;
3. Pour the olive oil inside a large saucepan and heat over medium heat. Add the onion and garlic for about five to eight minutes or until the onion is transparent;
4. Put the tomatoes, carrots, peppers and whisk to mix well in the blender or food processor;
5. Add the seasonings and a teaspoon to the pan of step 3. Add the shredded chicken, the mixture of step 4, the corn, the beans and 2/4 cup of cilantro. If you find the soup too thick, put water;

6. Cook with the pan partially covered for 30 minutes to an hour, until the corn stays soft;
7. Serve the soup decorated with the cheese and the rest of the coriander.

Nutritional Information

Calories Per Serving: 182

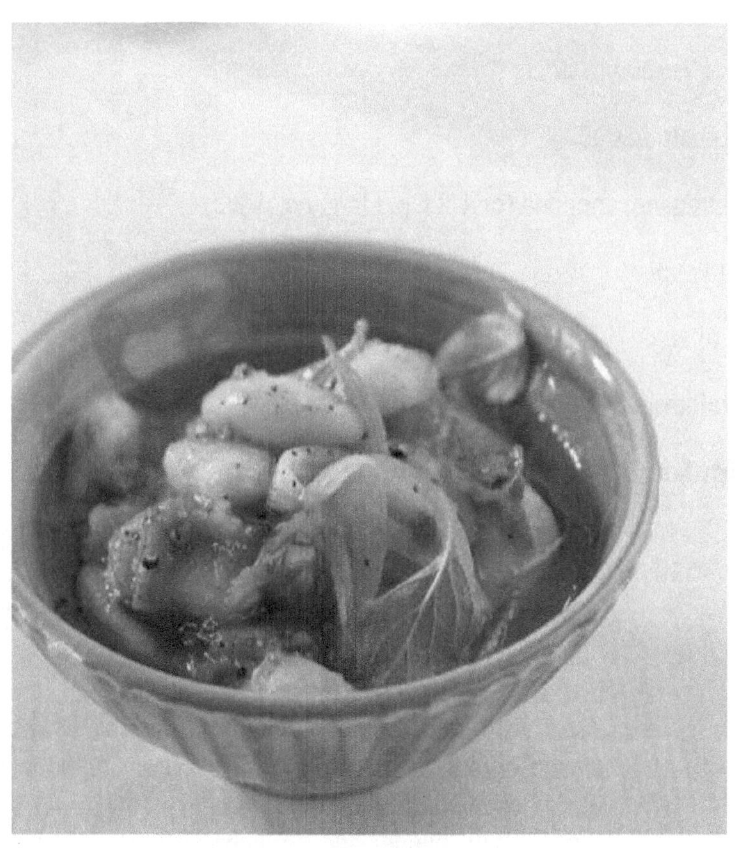

32.   Giant beans

Working time: 20 min.

Ingredients

For 2 servings

1 clove of garlic

1 onion

250 g of tomatoes

1 small can of giant white beans (225 g EW)

3 tbsp olive oil

125 ml of vegetable stock

1 tbsp tomato paste

1 tbsp. Oregano, chopped (or 1/2 tsp. Oregano, dried)

Salt and Pepper

1 pinch of sugar

Oregano leaves

Preparation

1. Finely chop 1 garlic clove. Cut 1 onion and 250 g of tomatoes into slices.
2. Rinse 1 small can of giant white beans (225 g EW) in a colander with cold water and drain.
3. Heat 3 tbsp olive oil. Fry the garlic and onions in a glassy sauce. Add tomatoes and saute briefly. Mix 125 ml of vegetable stock and 1 tbsp of tomato puree and pour. Season with 1 tablespoon of chopped oregano (or 1/2 Tl of dried oregano) salt, pepper and a pinch of sugar. Add beans and

heat for about 6-7 minutes. Serve decorated with oregano leaves.

Nutritional value

Per serving 284 kcal

Carbohydrates: 18 g

Protein: 10 g

Fat: 18 g

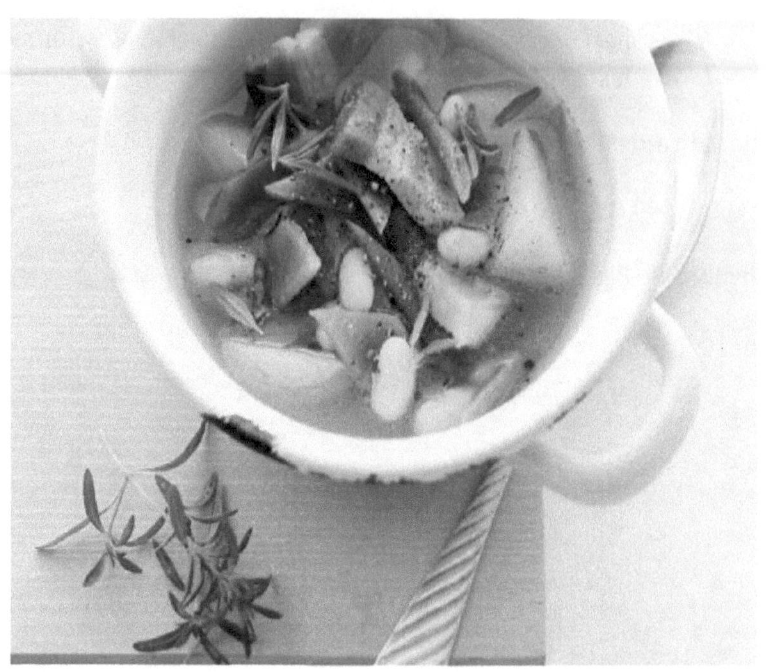

33. Stew with beans and bacon

Preparation: 25 min

Finished in 2 h 15 min

For 4 portions

Ingredients

800 grams meat-bone beef (chopped)

2 soup greens à 250 g

300 grams streaky

1 tbsp. butter

Salt

Pepper from the mill

2 bay leaves

600 grams firming new potatoes

2 spoons bacon grease

400 grams of flat beans

3 branches

Savoury

Preparation

1.   Rip off the meat bones. Wash, clean, and cut the birch trees. Heat the butter inside a saucepan and sauté the bacon grease in it, slightly browned. Approximately Drain 2 litres of cold water and add the bones. Bring to a boil and carefully scoop uprising foam. As soon as there is no more foam, put the greens in the pot and season with salt, pepper, and some bay leaves. Simmer at a moderate temperature for about 1.5 hours.

2.   In the meantime, wash the potatoes and roll them roughly. Wash the white beans inside a colander and drain. Wash and clean the flat beans and cut them diagonally into 4-5 cm pieces. Wash the savoury and pluck the leaves from the branches.

3.   Fish the bacon cubes out of the pot and put them aside. Remove the bones and greens; filter the broth through a kitchen towel. Bring to a boil inside a clean saucepan with the bacon and potatoes and cook for about 20 minutes till the potatoes are tender. Add the flat beans, the white beans, and the savoury in half the time. Season and serve in soup bowls.

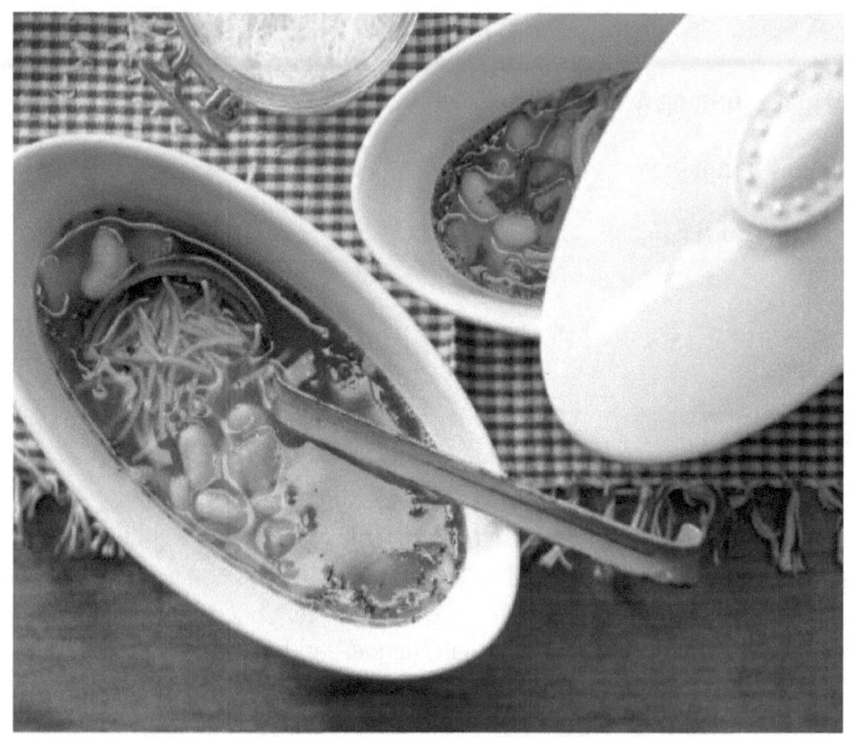

34.   Italian Noodle Bean Stew

With bacon and carrots

Italian noodle bean stew - Typical of Venetian cuisine: down-to-earth, hearty but not stressful

For 4 portions

Preparation: 50 min

Ingredients

1 can white beans (415 g sample)

3 small onions (about 150 g)

2 garlic cloves

2 spoons bacon grease

1 tbsp olive oil

800 ml classic vegetable broth

3 small carrots (about 200 g)

2 stems

Sage

Salt

Pepper

30 g parmesan cheese

225 g whole wheat vermicelli

Preparation

1.   Put beans in a sieve, rinse off with cold water and drain. Peel onions and garlic and finely dice.

2.   Heat the olive oil inside a saucepan, fry the bacon grease and onions in a glass oven while stirring slowly over medium heat.

3.   Add garlic and simmer for another 1 minute while stirring. Pour broth and bring to a boil.

4.   Wash carrots, peel and cut into 1 cm cubes. Add to the boiling broth and cook it at medium heat for 20 minutes.

5.   Wash the sage, shake dry, peel the leaves and finely chop, add the beans to the soup and cook for another 5 minutes. Season the soup with salt and pepper. Grate the parmesan finely.

6.   In the meantime, cook noodles in plenty of salted water according to the instructions in the pack, drain in a sieve and add to the soup just before serving. Serve with the freshly grated Parmesan. Who likes it creamier, mashed about half of the soup before the noodles come in, and gives the

puree back into the pot.

Nutritional Fact

Calories   377 kcal   (18%)

Protein   23 g   (23%)

Fat   9 g   (8th %)

Carbohydrates   49 g   (33%)

Added sugar   0 g   (0%)

Roughage   14 g   (47%)

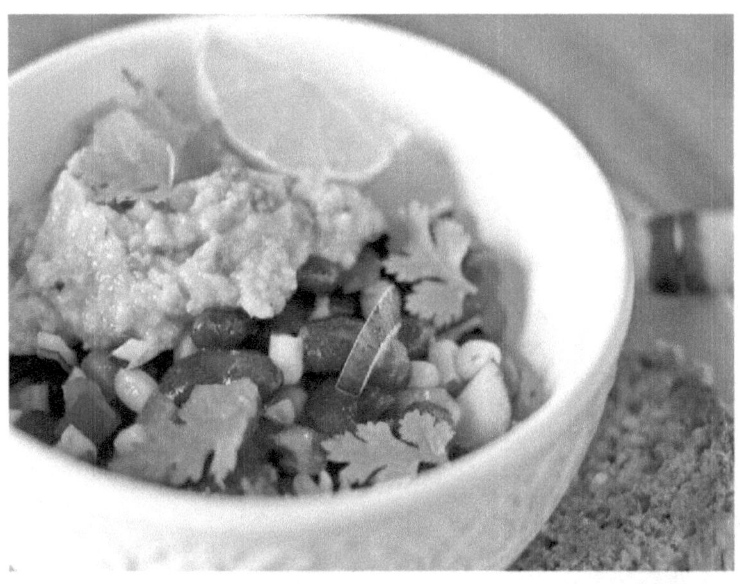

35.   Salad of red beans with guacamole

Homemade salad of red beans with guacamole makes a beautiful healthy plate! It's a vegetarian/vegan, gluten-free meal (if you want) that everyone will enjoy.

4 people

30 minutes

Ingredients for 4 people

1 unit (s) of Tomato (medium)

1 unit (s) of Onion (half onion purple)

1 unit (s) of red pepper (medium)

1 pinch of Pepper

1 unit (s) of Limón

1 pinch of salt

1 unit (s) of Green pepper

250 grams of Azuki a pot (canned red beans already cooked)

1 tablespoon of extra virgin olive oil

1 unit (s) of fresh Guacamole Frutas Montosa (Mercadona) you can make it homemade too

1 small cup of sweet corn in a can

Preparation

1. Prepare the salad by mixing all the chopped ingredients with the beans previously washed and drained.
2. Dress with lemon juice and oil and season with salt and pepper.
3. Serve the salad with the guacamole and toast with toasted bread.

Nutritional composition for 100 grs.

Composition   Amount (gr)   CDR (%)

Kcalories   353.04   18.4%

Carbohydrates   42.06   13.5

Proteins   14.75   30.8%

Fiber   13.82   46.1%

Fat   10.33   19.4%

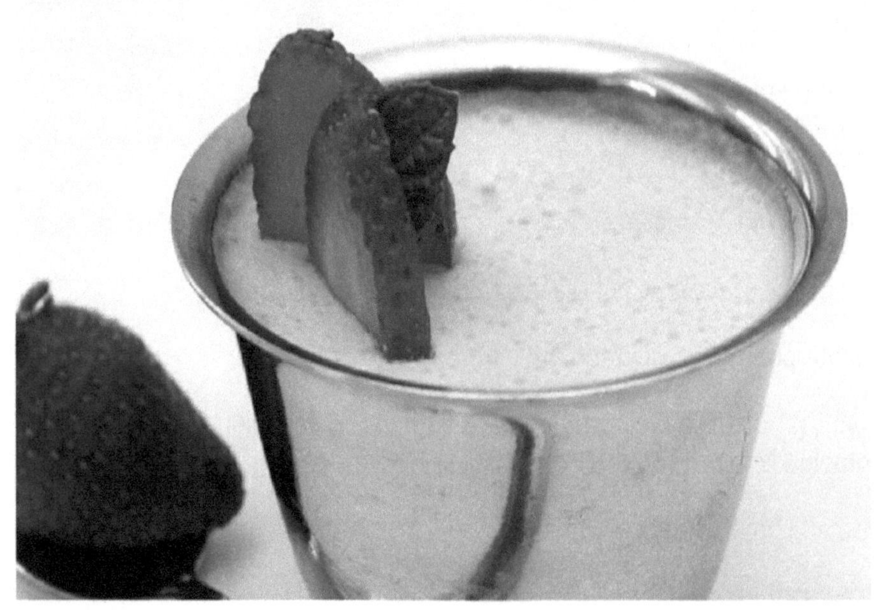

36. Homemade strawberry danonino recipe

Ingredients

120 g of water

3 or 4 strawberries

40 g of strawberry gelatin powder

200 g of cheese spread

100 g of liquid cream

20 g of sugar

Preparation

1. Heat the water 2 minutes, 100 degrees, speed 1.
2. We add the strawberries and grind for 8 seconds at speed 7.
3. Add the gelatin and mix 1 minute at speed 3.
4. Finally add the cheese, cream, and sugar in this order and mix 30 seconds at progressive speed 5-7-9
5. Pour the mixture of the homemade strawberry danonine into individual cups and let stand 3 hours in the fridge.

Traditional:

Grind the strawberries with the help of a blender. Strain if we consider it necessary.

Add the cream, sugar, and cheese to the strawberries. Mix well and reserve.

Heat the water inside a saucepan till it starts to boil. Add the strawberry puree and gelatin. Allow to cook over medium heat for a couple of minutes, stirring constantly, so it does not catch.

Divide the mixture into individual cups and let stand in the refrigerator for 3 hours.

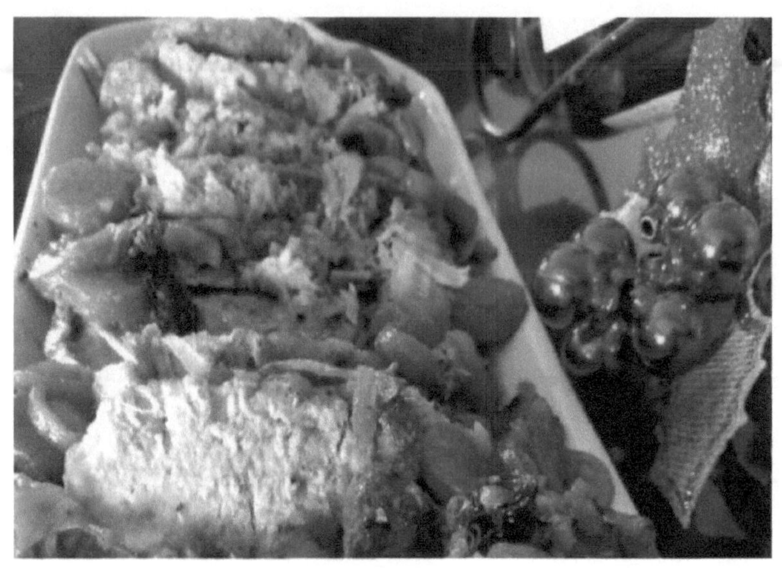

37.   Pickled Pork Loin Recipe

8 people

2h 30m

Ingredients:

1 pork loin

1 kilo of carrots

1 and 1/2 onion

Garlic

Black pepper in grain

Olive oil

 Sour orange juice

Vinegar

2 cups of water

Herbs of smell (thyme, laurel, and oregano)

Bobbin (for accompaniment)

Preparation

1. The loin is marinated with garlic, salt, pepper, and orange juice, and left to rest for about four hours.
2. It is the meat fried to seal on both sides.
3. Then add carrots (5 sliced carrots), 1 onion and herbs (laurel, thyme, and oregano) to taste.
4. Now you put two cups of water, 1 large garlic and salt, cover the pot (remember that preferably we are going to make the sirloin pickled in pot express) and cook about 20 minutes.
5. Is the solution prepared pork loin: 6 carrots and 1 onion are cut and fried in olive oil with garlic in a pan.
6. It is cooked with water, a little vinegar, and herbs odor and is added four balls of black pepper.
7. As the last step, slices of loin are added to the pickle, and then they are left to soak for some minutes before serving the pork in vinegar accompanied by white bread type bolillo.
8. Serve the freshly made pickled pork tenderloin.

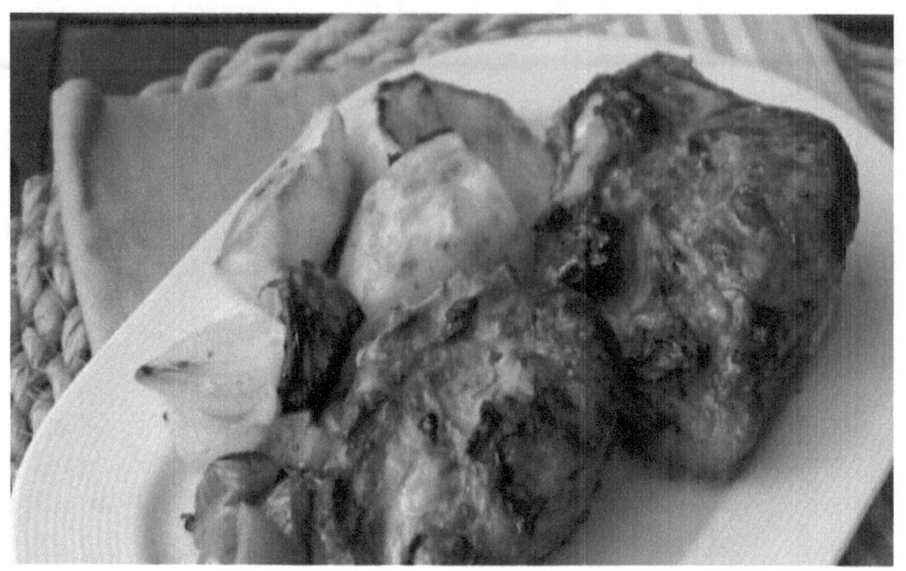

38. Pork cheeks recipe baked.

4 people

1h 30m

Ingredients:

4 pork lanes

2 onions

4 tomatoes

4 potatoes

6 cloves of garlic

200 milliliters of white wine

1 pinch of pepper

1 pinch of salt

1 jet of olive oil

1 pinch of parsley

Preparation

1. We prepare the ingredients to start making the baked pork cheeks.
2. We put the cheeks in a fountain; we make some cuts in each one in the form of a cross.
3. In a mortar we chop the garlic with a little parsley, add the white wine and a little water.
4. With the mince we have prepared of garlic and wine, we season the cheeks, which are well soaked. We booked a bit of the picada. We salt and put a little pepper. We cover the fountain and let rest for an hour.
5. Trick: If we put the Cordilleras with bone in the oven, it will be more tasty than boned since the meat that stays closest to the bone is always the tastiest.
6. After this time, we put the meat in a baking dish with all the dressing it takes, cut the onions into quarters, the tomatoes and the potatoes sliced in half. Sprinkle everything with the rest of the bite that we have left and a stream of olive oil. We put the cheeks baked in the oven at 180 °C. We will go around the meat so that it is browned for everything. The cooking time will vary according to the size of the cheeks.

Tip: If the tray is dry, we will add water.

When we see that they are well browned, and the tender potatoes turn off the oven. And the baked pork cheeks will be ready to eat.

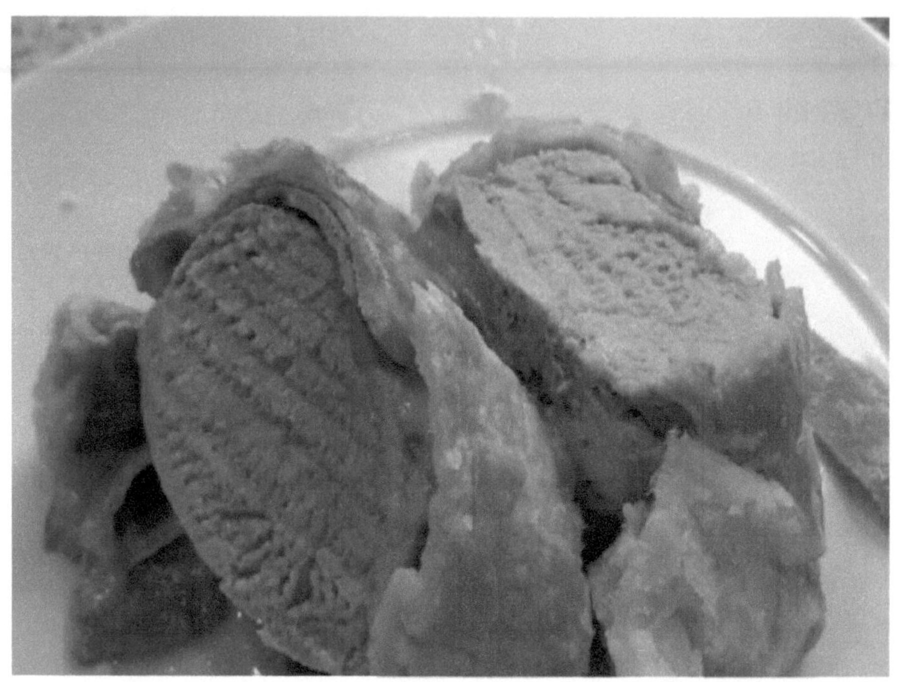

39.   Recipe of Pork tenderloin with baked puff pastry

For 6 guests

Cooking time: 45m

Ingredients:

1 sheet of puff pastry

1 fillet of pork

6 slices of bacon

6 slices of cheese

1 egg to paint

Preparation

1. We preheat the oven to 220 ° C. We pepper the sirloin and

seal it by passing it through a frying pan. We reserve and let cool.

2. Stretch the puff pastry sheet. We divide the sheet mentally into 3, and in the central section, we place the slices of cheese and then the slices of bacon in such a way that they then wrap the sirloin.

3. Once the tenderloin is tempered (so that it does not soften the puff pastry), place it on the bacon. We passed the slices over the sirloin so that it is covered and we obtain a pork tenderloin wrapped in bacon.

4. Finally, we close the puff pastry. Spread the pork tenderloin wrapped in puff pastry with the beaten egg and put in the oven for about 30 minutes.

5. We take out, let cool a little, cut and enjoy this delicious pork tenderloin with baked puff pastry!

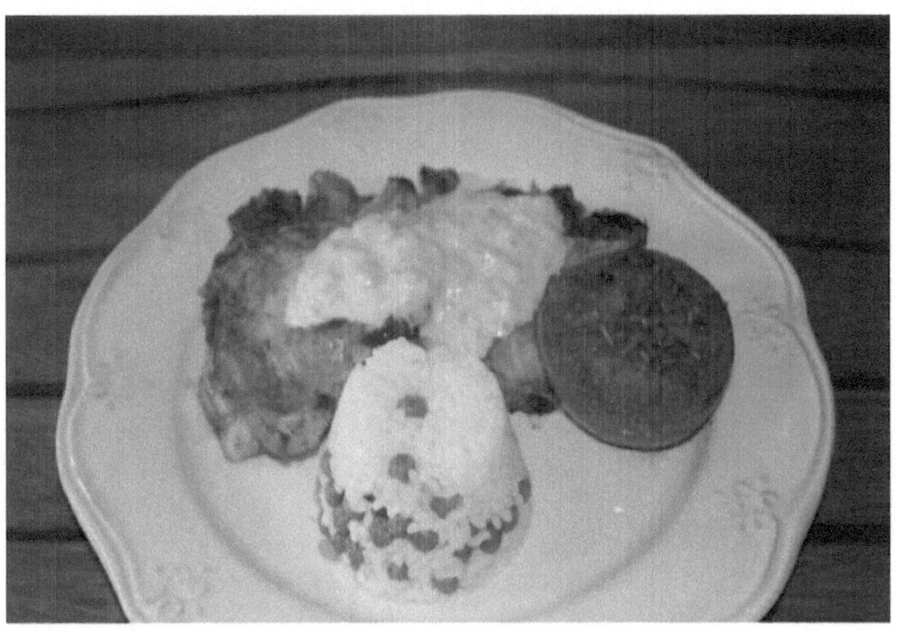

40.   Recipe for Pork Chops in an Easy Sauce

For 4 guests

Cooking time: 45m

Ingredients:

4 pork chops

1 tablespoon of olive oil

2 large tomatoes cut in half

1 tablespoon chopped chives

Ingredient for onion sauce:

1 pinch of ground clove

25 grams of butter

25 grams of flour

200 milliliters of cream or milk cream

1 pinch of ground black pepper

½ teaspoon of salt

2 onions

Preparation

1. Heat the oil inside a large skillet, season with the chops and fry over low heat for about 5 minutes.
2. We turn them over and add the tomatoes cut in half and sprinkled with cloves — Fry for ten more minutes.
3. While they are making the chops, we are preparing the onion sauce. In a pan put the butter to heat and in it fry the onion very chopped, and when it is turning golden brown, add the flour and a low heat stirring for one or two minutes.

4. Withdraw from the heat and add the cream or cream, season, put back to the fire and wait until the sauce to accompany chops boil without stirring, about 3 minutes to achieve a thick and smooth sauce.
5. We put stewed pork chops and tomatoes in a serving dish. The onion sauce is sprinkled over the meat, and the tomatoes are sprinkled with chopped chives.
6. This recipe has accompanied this recipe of pork chops in an easy sauce with cooked white.

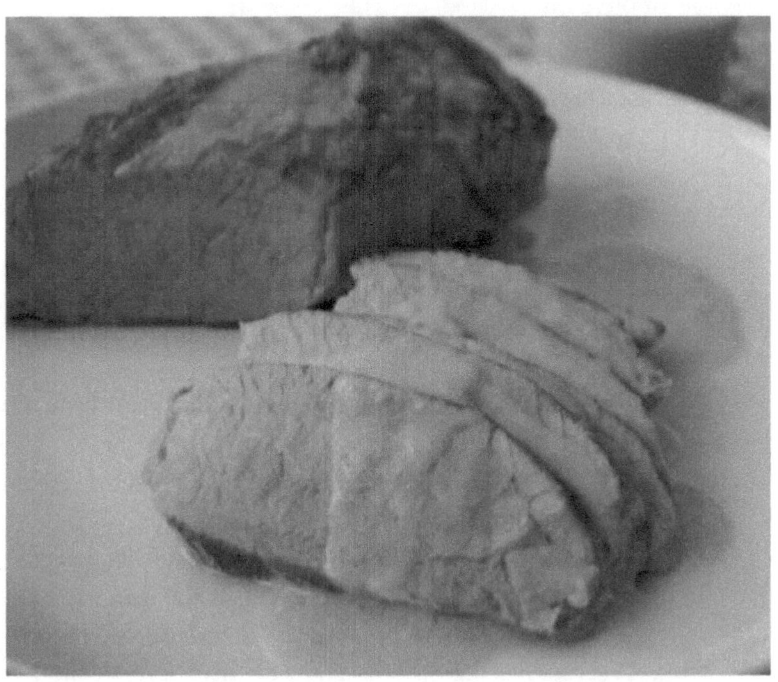

41.   Recipe for Pork Tenderloin in Parmesan Sauce

For 6 guests

Cooking time: 45m

Ingredients:

2 sirloins

60 grams of Parmesan cheese

200 milliliters of cream for cooking or cream of milk

100 milliliters of milk

1 pinch of salt

1 pinch of pepper

4 tablespoons of olive oil

Preparation

1. We clean the sirloins from the sheets and fat, season and brown them in a pan with the 4 tablespoons of oil over high heat. It must brown well on the outside.
2. Meanwhile, we grate the Parmesan cheese. As said, if you prefer you can substitute this cheese for another you like, although it is one of the protagonists of the sirloin recipe in cheese sauce.
3. We are going around the sirloins to let them brown on all sides.
4. When they are golden brown, add the cream or cream. Let cook over medium heat for about 5 minutes.
5. We put the grated Parmesan cheese, and let it cook until there is a sauce; We tried the salt. If the sauce is too thick, we can pour milk to our liking. We turn off and let cool.
6. We remove the sirloins and cut them into steaks to serve them.
7. Once cut into steaks, we will put them in the casserole again. At the time of serving, we give a heat stroke and enjoy this exquisite recipe of pork tenderloin in a parmesan sauce. This dish is ideal for parties or family meals, accompanied by a good salad or baked potatoes.

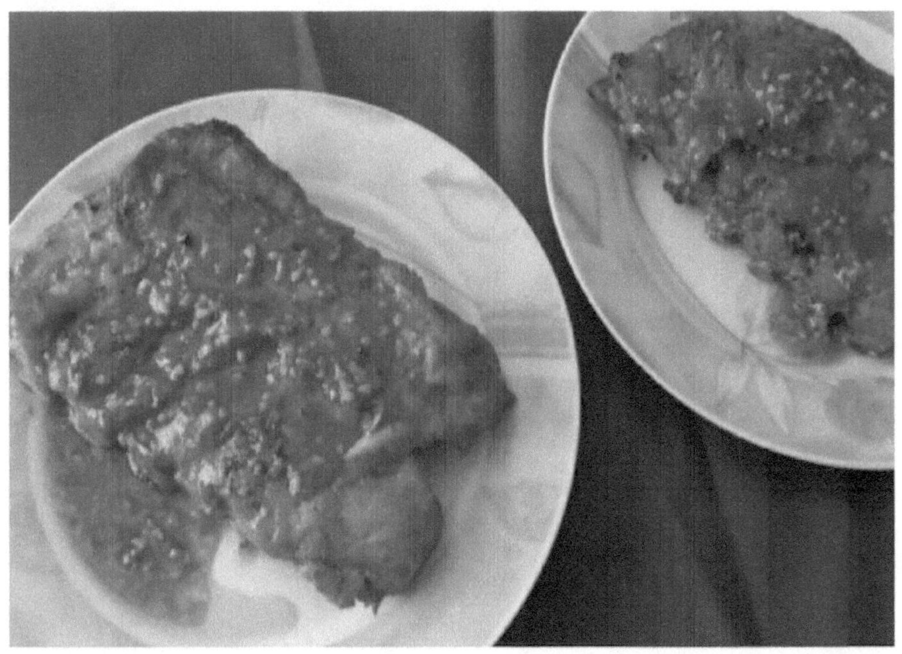

42.   **Recipe for Pork Ribs baked with garlic and parsley**

For 2 people

1h 30m

Ingredients:

1 rack of pork of 1 kg

1 head of garlic

2 branches of fresh parsley

1 teaspoon salt

2 tablespoons of extra virgin olive oil

1 small glass of white wine

1 pinch of ground cumin

1 pinch of ground black pepper

Preparation

1. We split the ribs into two halves of approximately the same size. We place them in a wide source and reserve.
2. Peel the garlic and chop it together with the parsley. We reserved a moment, and we continued preparing the rest of the ingredients of the recipe of ribs with garlic and parsley.
3. Season the ribs on each side with a pinch of pepper and cumin.
4. Divide the garlic and the chopped parsley over the ribs and water with a trickle of olive oil. Add salt to taste and pour white wine to enhance the flavor of baked pork ribs with garlic and parsley.
5. Cover and let stand several hours for the meat to take the dressings so, if you can rest a whole night much better.
6. Place the meat in a dish suitable for baking when we go to bake the ribs and pour the liquid. We introduce in the oven preheated to 180 °C, and we bake until the meat is at the point that we like. The time depends on each oven and each rack, but it will oscillate between 30 and 60 minutes.
7. We can serve the baked pork ribs with garlic and parsley accompanied by a light salad, such as lettuce with orange salad , or a few potatoes and we will have a complete meal. Enjoy your meal!

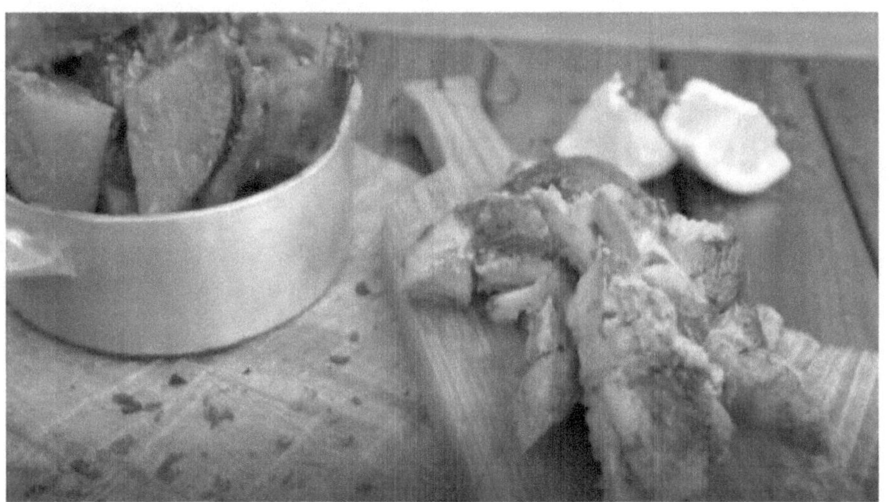

43.   Braided Pork Roulade

Ingredients

400 gr. of pork matambre

4 garlics cut in half

1 tbsp of oregano

1 tbsp of ground chili

C / n olive

2 sweet potatoes

2 tbsp of shortening

1 tbsp made of olives

1 glass of dark beer

1/4 cup of milk cream

Salt, pepper, and lemon

C / n lard

Preparation

1. Cut three strips of the matambre without reaching the end of one of the tips, season with salt, pepper, ground aji, oregano and a touch of olive. Take 30 minutes to marinate in the refrigerator.
2. Wrap the sweet potatoes with a touch of butter and bring them directly to the embers until they are ready. Cut into pieces and bring to a pan with a touch of butter, add the black beer, let the alcohol evaporate, unite with a touch of cream and season.
3. Remove the slaughter, assemble the braided by adding a few cloves of garlic inside, and bring to cook over high heat 7 minutes per side.

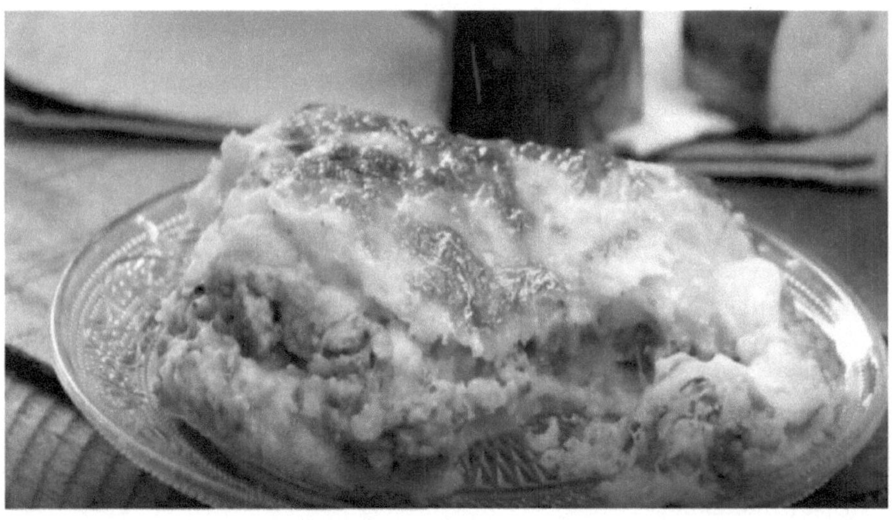

44.   Banana Pie and Pork

Ingredients

For the bananas:

5 ripe bananas cut into slices

A few squirts of oil for frying

3 tablespoons of butter

Sprinkle sugar

For the meat:

A few squirts of olive oil

1 spoonful of the achiote

½ chopped onion

½ chopped sweet pepper

1 chopped Panamanian chile

4 cloves of garlic, chopped

½ tomatos in cubes

2 cups ground pork

A ½ cup of raisins

A pinch of cumin

1 teaspoon garlic powder

Salt and pepper

A pinch of sugar

For the filling:

2 cups ground beans

2 cups of custard

3 cups of cheese

Preparation

1. Boil the bananas until they are well cooked, peeled and in a food processor mix until you get a puree.
2. In a bowl, stir the banana puree with half Turrialba cheese and salt to taste. Reserve.
3. In a pan over medium heat, heat the oil and fry the chili and onion.
4. Add the ground beef, the whole seasoning, and the ranchera sauce. Mix until the meat is well cooked — salt and pepper to taste.
5. Inside a baking dish, place half of the banana puree, then add the ground beans, one layer of the meat and another of puree.
6. Top with the mozzarella cheese and the rest of Turrialba type cheese.
7. Take to the oven for 15 minutes at 180 degrees until the cheese is browned.

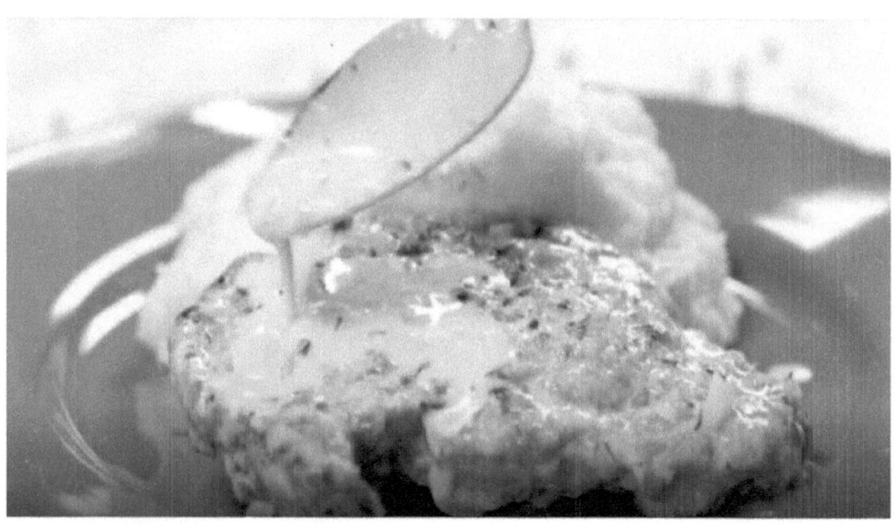

45.   Pork Chops with Cream

Preparation:

Prep time30 min

Cooking time30 min

Serving time4

Ingredients

4 pork ribs (chops)

½ cup flour

1 tbsp. of garlic powder

1 tbsp. onion powder

4 tbsps. of butter

¼ cup of white wine

¼ cup of lemon juice

1 tbsp. lemon zest

3 cloves garlic, chopped

1 tbsp. from thyme

½ cup of cream

1 tbsp. of chopped red onion

Salt and pepper

Mashed potatoes to accompany

Preparation

1. In a refractory combine flour, garlic powder, onion powder and season. Mix well.
2. To pass ribs on this preparation on both sides.

3. Inside a pan, melt 2 tablespoons of butter and bring the chops to seal on both sides. Remove.
4. In the same pan, deglaze the bottom with white wine, lemon juice, lemon zest, thyme, chopped garlic, chopped onion and the remaining two spoons of butter. Let it melt and incorporate the cream. Incorporate all
5. Flavors
6. Reattach the ribs and salsear.

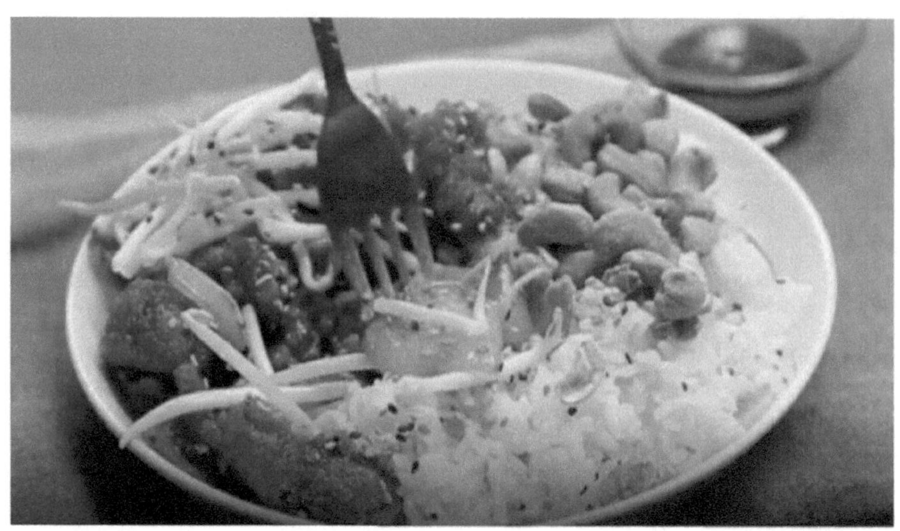

46. Bittersweet Pig

Ingredients

1/2 red bell

1/2 green bell

1 onion

1/4 cabbage (if it is hakusai better, but white)

500 gr. of pork carré without bone

200 gr. of bean sprouts

1 lt. of neutral oil

Sweet and sour sauce 300ml (sweet chili)

50 gr. of sugar

50 ml. of soy sauce

Garlic 2 teeth

1 ginger tooth

50 gr. of toasted cashews

Preparation

For the pig:

1. Season the pork with soy, garlic, ginger, and sugar.
2. In a bowl with cornstarch, coat the pork bites until they are completely white, without sticking between them.
3. Pour into a fryer with oil at approx. 170° for 7 minutes or until they take a slightly golden color.

For vegetables:

1. Pour three tablespoons of oil into the wok and bring to maximum heat.
2. Sauté the morrón and the onion until they soften.
3. Once the vegetables soften, pour the cabbage, the pork, and sauté for 1 minute.
4. After the minute, season with Sweet and Sour Sauce until you reach the desired point.
5. Once everything is dyed pink/red, serve in a deep dish, and decorate with cashews and bean sprouts.

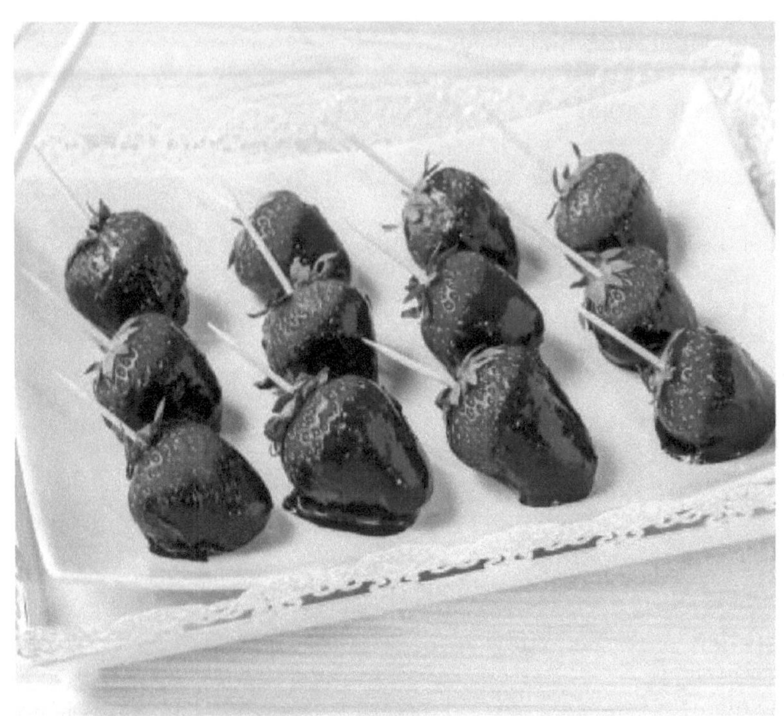

47. Crunchy Chocolate Covered Strawberries

Share this dish with a loved one as a special treat or treat yourself to something good with this simple dessert!

Servings: 2

Preparation time: 10 mins

Cooking time: 10 mins

Nutritional Fact: Carbohydrates: 12g

Ingredients

10 fresh strawberries

1 Atkins crispy milk chocolate bar

Preparation

1. Lay out a baking tray, including baking paper. Break the Atkins bar into even pieces and place it in a heat-resistant bowl (take one that fits your pot).
2. Fill a pot 1/3 with water; bring the water to a boil. Once cooked, reduce the heat. Place the bowl over the pot - make sure the bowl does not come into contact with the water. Mix the chocolate using a metal spoon until completely melted and smooth.
3. Dip each strawberry about 2/3 into the melted chocolate, keeping it at the top, then place it on the baking paper. Repeat for all strawberries.
4. Put the strawberries in the fridge to cool.
5. Use the remaining chocolate to decorate your platter.

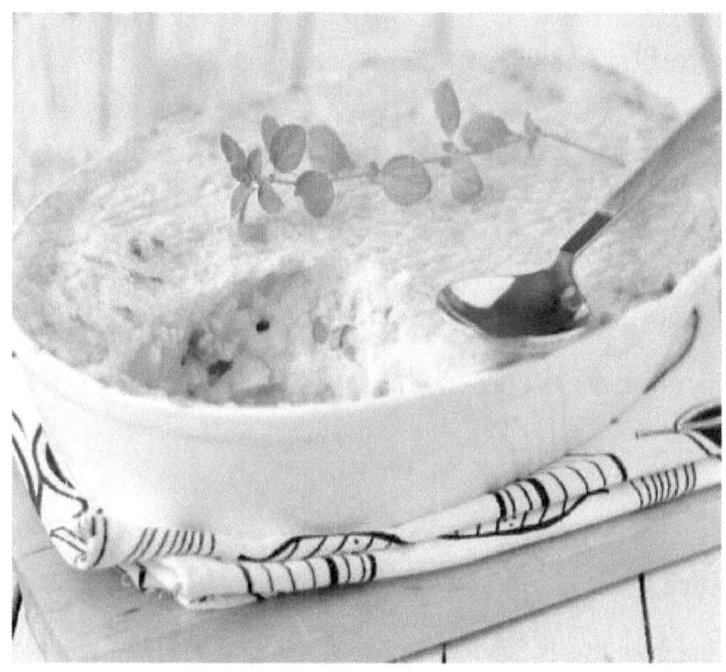

48.   Fish pie

Fancy a delicious fish cake? Try this recipe with some salmon, white fish, tomatoes and spices. A great meal to prepare for a cozy dinner with friends. Healthy and naturally low carb.

Servings: 4

Preparation time: 10 mins

Cooking time: 60 minutes

Nutritional Fact: Carbohydrates: 5g

Ingredients

1 tablespoon of olive oil

50 grams of white onion

2 cloves of garlic

400 grams of canned tomatoes

1 tablespoon of fresh ginger

1 teaspoon of cinnamon powder

1 teaspoon salt

1 teaspoon of black pepper

150 grams of salmon fillet

150 grams of white fish fillet

2 tablespoons butter

100 grams of celery

Preparation

Preheat the oven to gas level 3 or 175 ° C. Chop the celery and cook for 7 -
10 minutes in salted water. Pass, purée, and mix in the butter. Taste it with
salt and pepper. Put the fish in a pot of boiling water, with just enough water
to cover it. Cook for 5 minutes. The fish should be dark and easily
disintegrate. Drain the fish and put it in a bowl. Put the oil in a pan over
medium heat and sweat the onion and garlic for 5 minutes. Stir in the boiled
fish, chopped tomatoes, cinnamon, ginger, salt, and pepper. Let it simmer

over medium heat to allow the flavours to develop. Put the mass in a small frying pan and cover with the puree. Cook everything inside the oven for 20 minutes, until the puree is crispy.

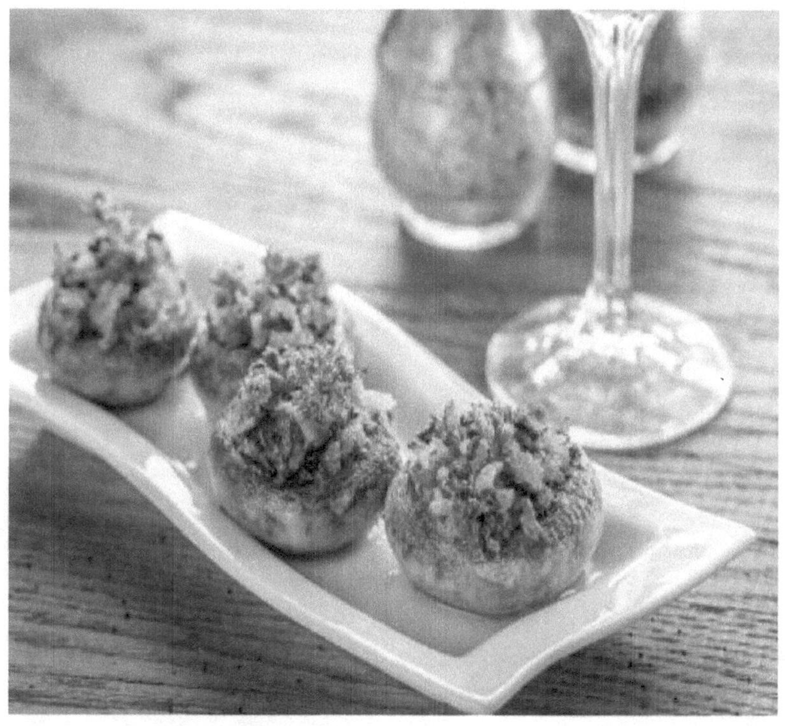

49.   Sausages Stuffed Mushrooms

Servings: 1

Preparation time: 10 mins

Cooking time: 25 minutes

Nutritional Fact: Carbohydrates:6g

Ingredients

2 sausages

1 clove of garlic

2 tablespoons cream cheese

1 tablespoon of ground flaxseed

1/2 onion

Share page

Preparation

Remove the intestines and fry the sausage with the pressed garlic. Then place it on the page for later. Then remove the stems of mushrooms and chop them small. Mix the finely chopped champignon stems with the cream cheese and then add the cooled sausage meat. Finally, add the ground flax seeds and fill the mushrooms with the mixture. Place the mushrooms in a large casserole dish and bake at 160 ° C for 25 minutes.

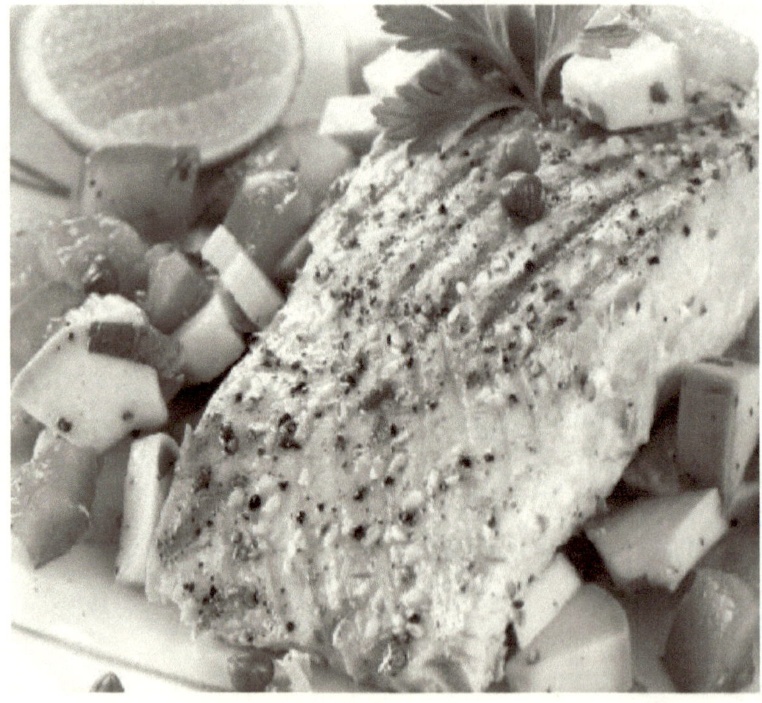

50.   Salmon with avocado salsa
Servings: 1

Preparation time: 10 mins

Cooking time: 15 minutes

Nutritional Fact: Carbohydrates: 5g

Ingredients

0.5 tablespoon olive oil

0.25 teaspoon salt

0.5 teaspoon black pepper

0.5 teaspoon paprika powder

115 grams of salmon fillet

0.5 Avocado

0.25 red onions

1 tablespoon of fresh lime juice

1 tablespoon of fresh coriander

3 cherry tomatoes

Preparation

1. Mix the oil, salt, pepper including paprika into a bowl. Coat the salmon fillet including the marinade and put it in the fridge for 30 minutes. Grate the salmon on both sides for two minutes over high heat.
2. Mix the avocado, chopped tomatoes, 1/4 red onion, the juice of a lime, 1 tablespoon of olive oil including salt to taste in a separate bowl. Serve the salmon on the avocado salsa and garnish with chopped cilantro. Serve with a mixed green salad.

If you're searching for a diet that can accelerate fat burning and weight loss and at the same time help your health, intermittent fasting may be the method you are looking for.

In addition to accelerating weight loss and fat burning, other benefits of intermittent fasting can be listed as regulating blood sugar, protecting your brain, protecting heart health and reducing inflammation.

There are many various methods of intermittent fasting, which can adapt to different lifestyles. You can try different methods to find the method that suits you best.

Intermittent fasting may not be fitting for everyone, especially people with certain health problems. However, for many people, it can be an important part of healthy living.